SYMPOSIA OF THE SECTION ON MICROBIOLOGY
THE NEW YORK ACADEMY OF MEDICINE

Number 3

THE PATHOGENESIS AND PATHOLOGY OF VIRAL DISEASES

THE PATHOGENESIS AND PATHOLOGY OF VIRAL DISEASES

EDITED BY

John G. Kidd

SYMPOSIUM HELD AT THE
NEW YORK ACADEMY OF MEDICINE
DECEMBER 14 and 15, 1948

1950 New York
COLUMBIA UNIVERSITY PRESS

COPYRIGHT 1950 NEW YORK
COLUMBIA UNIVERSITY PRESS

PUBLISHED IN GREAT BRITAIN,
CANADA, AND INDIA
BY GEOFFREY CUMBERLEGE
OXFORD UNIVERSITY PRESS,
LONDON, TORONTO, AND BOMBAY

MANUFACTURED IN THE UNITED STATES OF AMERICA

SECTION ON MICROBIOLOGY
THE NEW YORK ACADEMY OF MEDICINE

Officers
GREGORY SCHWARTZMAN, *Chairman*
HARRY MOST, *Secretary*

Advisory Board
JOHN G. KIDD
RENÉ J. DUBOS
FRANK L. HORSFALL, JR.
COLIN M. MACLEOD
RALPH S. MUCKENFUSS

Organizing Committee for Symposium Number 3
JOHN G. KIDD, *Chairman*
RALPH S. MUCKENFUSS
GREGORY SHWARTZMAN

Foreword

ON MAY 1, 1947, the Fellowship of The New York Academy of Medicine approved the organization of the Section on Microbiology, thus establishing the first section of the Academy devoted to basic medical sciences.

Ample opportunities are already available for presentation and publication of scientific papers. However, with increasing diversity, complexity, and specialization, there is evident a need for opportunity to digest and correlate the rapidly accumulating body of new knowledge. The main objectives of the new Section are to provide a forum for the exchange of information amongst the workers engaged in basic and clinical sciences.

Accordingly, the scope of interest of the Section on Microbiology is broadly defined, as embodying the following: (1) bacteriology, mycology and parasitology; (2) viruses and rickettsiae; (3) maladies of unknown or uncertain etiology, possibly of infectious origin; (4) immunology; (5) chemotherapy; (6) pathology relative to microbiology; and (7) methods of study adopted from related sciences, as applied to microbiology. The programs of meetings of the Section are arranged to deal with single topics in their various aspects. In addition to regular monthly evening meetings, several symposia are organized yearly, each consisting of consecutive afternoon and evening sessions. The participants present extensive reviews in their particular fields of endeavor, thus bringing correlated and authoritative scientific data and concepts to the attention of the microbiologists and allied laboratory and clinical investigators. Unpublished symposia are soon forgotten, but their benefits may be retained by prompt publication. Important service is rendered by the Columbia University Press which has undertaken the publication of this series under the auspices of the New York Academy of Medicine and the editorship of the respective chairmen of the symposia.

GREGORY SHWARTZMAN

Contents

1. INTRODUCTION 3
   JOHN C. KIDD

2. THE SPREAD OF VIRUSES FROM INFECTED TO SUSCEPTIBLE HOSTS 6
   RICHARD E. SHOPE, *Department of Animal and Plant Pathology of The Rockefeller Institute for Medical Research*

3. THE CULTURE AND EFFECTS OF VIRUSES IN CHICK EMBRYO CELLS 19
   C. JOHN BUDDINGH, *Louisiana State University School of Medicine*

4. THE RELATIONSHIPS OF VIRUSES AND CELLS, WITH PARTICULAR REFERENCE TO THE INTERFERENCE PHENOMENON 31
   GILBERT DALLDORF, *Division of Laboratories and Research, New York State Department of Health*

5. THE ACTIVATORS OF VIRUSES BY ADSORPTION COFACTORS 47
   THOMAS F. ANDERSON, *Johnson Foundation, University of Pennsylvania*

6. THE ELECTRON MICROSCOPIC STUDY OF VIRUS GROWTH 62
   RALPH W. G. WYCKOFF, *Laboratory of Physical Biology, Experimental Biology and Medicine Institute, National Institutes of Health*

7. PATHOLOGY AND PATHOGENESIS OF THE CUTANEOUS LESIONS OF VARIOLA, VACCINIA, HERPES SIMPLEX, HERPES ZOSTER, AND VARICELLA 73
   T. F. MCNAIR SCOTT, H. BLANK, L. L. CORIELL, and H. CROUSE, *Department of Pediatrics, The Children's Hospital of*

Philadelphia, and Department of Dermatology and Syphilology and Department of Medicine, University of Pennsylvania

8. PATHOGENESIS OF THE VIRAL EXANTHEMS AS EXEMPLIFIED BY MOUSE POX (INFECTIOUS ECTROMELIA) OF MICE 99
FRANK FENNER, Walter and Eliza Hall Institute, Melbourne, Australia, and The Rockefeller Institute for Medical Research

9. CARDIAC LESIONS PRODUCED BY VIRUSES 107
JOHN M. PEARCE, Department of Pathology, Long Island College of Medicine, Hoagland Laboratory, and Departments of Pathology and Surgery, Cornell University Medical College, The New York Hospital–Cornell Medical Center

10. PATHOLOGY OF YELLOW FEVER 134
J. E. ASH, Former Scientific Director, American Registry of Pathology, Army Institute of Pathology, Washington, D. C.

11. REACTIONS OF THE CELLS OF THE RESPIRATORY TRACT TO VIRUS INFECTIONS 153
THOMAS P. MAGILL, Department of Microbiology and Immunology, Long Island College of Medicine

12. PROLIFERATIVE LESIONS CAUSED BY VIRUSES AND VIRUS-LIKE AGENTS 161
JOHN C. KIDD, Department of Pathology, The New York Hospital–Cornell Medical Center

13. THE PATHOLOGY OF LYMPHATIC CHORIOMENINGITIS VIRUS INFECTION: A DISCUSSON 181
R. D. LILLIE, National Institutes of Health

14. THE PATHOLOGY OF SOME VIRAL ENCEPHALITIDES 194
ABNER WOLF, Departments of Pathology and Neurology, Columbia University College of Physicians and Surgeons and the Neurological Institute of New York

15. THE NATURE AND PATHOGENESIS OF NEURONAL CHANGES IN POLIOMYELITIS 214
HOWARD A. HOWE, Poliomyelitis Research Center, Department of Epidemiology, Johns Hopkins University

THE PATHOGENESIS AND PATHOLOGY
OF VIRAL DISEASES

Chapter 1

INTRODUCTION

By John G. Kidd

OUR KNOWLEDGE of viruses and the diseases they cause is both wide and useful. Already consequential in Jenner's time, it received great impetus from his memorable translation into science of what had for some time been dairy folklore; later it was influenced by Pasteur's successes, and notably by his failure on repeated attempts to cultivate a bacterium causative of rabies. After Iwanowski's demonstration in 1892 and Beijerinck's in 1898, that a "living contagious fluid" is responsible for mosaic disease of tobacco plants, Loeffler and Frosch found that a similar agent causes foot-and-mouth disease in animals. Then in rapid succession other investigators began to perceive that agents of this kind—now called filtrable viruses—are widely prevalent in nature. Facts about these pathogens and their effects have steadily accumulated ever since, so that today the physician at the bedside and his colleague in the laboratory have at hand the means of determining case by case that viruses cause a number of serious and prevalent diseases in man—smallpox, chicken pox, measles, poliomyelitis, yellow fever, influenza, and the common cold, to mention but a few. In addition, knowledge equally definite and beneficial has been gained from a study of other viruses which in the aggregate cause staggering economic losses in animals and plants and which in some instances also threaten the health of human beings.

Fortunately indeed, we have gone beyond the mere isolation of these powerful pathogens and the recognition of the diseases they produce. Thus the prevention of smallpox has for a century and a half required only the sensible and diligent application of Jenner's teachings, while the threat of yellow fever has long been held in check by watchful control over the insect vectors responsible for its spread, and its conquest is now doubly assured by the availability of a vaccine laboriously cultured for its prevention. Furthermore, a number of other viral diseases in man, animals, and plants can likewise be controlled by preventive measures, and recently the prospect has begun to appear that chemotherapeutic agents may be found which will act against viruses even after they have begun to exert their ill effects on cells.

And this is by no means all. For studies on the nature and effects of filtrable viruses have extended knowledge in numerous directions and have provided problems of enduring interest and intellectual stimulation to a wide variety of biologists: to the bacteriologists, now become microbiologists, who discovered the agents and found that they pass through filters which hold bacteria back, and that while the viruses all fail to grow on lifeless media, some of them will propagate freely in association with living cells cultured *in vitro;* to the immunologists, who observed that infection with a filtrable virus gives rise characteristically to an immunity that may be lasting and is often accompanied by specific antibodies in the blood of the immune host and by an altered reactivity of his tissues to the virus and its products, and who continue to seek and find effective ways of stimulating antiviral immunity by artificial means; to the pathologists, who have learned much about the characteristic and harmful effects produced by viruses in the cells they prey upon; to the biophysicists, who have devised means of visualizing the viruses and of measuring their sizes, shapes, and densities; to the biochemists, who have isolated a number of the agents in more or less purified state and whose work has made it plain that the nucleoproteins are prominent amongst the substances comprising them; and, finally, to the geneticists and cytologists, who have lately begun to see in the viruses the simplest of available things that follow hereditary patterns as they grow and change.

Yet much remains to be learned about the viruses, and even more about their effects on cells. This is all too plain to those workers who have long studied the viruses by means of diverse techniques in the laboratory without as yet approaching an understanding of their origin, nature, and mode of reproduction. It is no whit less manifest to all who have had firsthand experience with viral diseases at the bedside, notably to those physicians who have lived through epidemics of poliomyelitis while ignorant of its pathogenesis and powerless to forestall or remedy the effects of its causative virus, and to those clinical investigators who, while appalled at the actual and potential

INTRODUCTION

harmfulness of viruses responsible for the common respiratory infections, must point without pride to the hiatuses remaining in our knowledge of them. With the aim of probing into the unknown as well as reviewing what is known about the pathogenesis and pathology of certain viral infections, this symposium has been arranged.

Chapter 2

THE SPREAD OF VIRUSES FROM INFECTED TO SUSCEPTIBLE HOSTS

By RICHARD E. SHOPE, *Department of Animal and Plant Pathology of the Rockefeller Institute for Medical Research*

I HOPE that I have not interpreted the title assigned me too broadly, because I do not intend to try to outline, for instance, just how the measles virus or the mumps virus gets from Johnny Jones to Mary Smith. Instead, I am going to endeavor to shed a little indirect light on that phase of virus epidemiology which appears to be shunned by most orthodox epidemiologists, namely, the question of the origin of the virus responsible for infecting the "first cases" in an outbreak and its possible whereabouts between outbreaks. Strictly speaking, this is within the scope of my subject because the title does not stipulate that the infected host must be in the same epidemic as the susceptible host to which it spreads its virus. I am going to limit my discussion to pointing out a few things that we know about the inception of outbreaks of certain virus diseases among animals and let this material serve as possible food for your thoughts in connection with human virus diseases problems. I have chosen to discuss animal rather than human virus diseases because the animal conditions are more amenable to the experimental approach, because they are less complicated by the influence of extraneous factors such as mechanized travel, mass immunization, psychological factors, and the like, and because I am personally more familiar with them than I am with the human virus diseases as a group.

Consideration of the natural history of an outbreak of an animal virus disease frequently gives a clue as to the origin of the virus responsible for the "first case." I should just like briefly to give a few known facts about certain virus diseases of animals which illustrate what I mean. In some of the examples to be cited, the epidemiology is understood; in others it remains to be worked out. The examples are as follows:

THE SPREAD OF VIRUSES

HOG CHOLERA

Hog cholera is a virus disease which during the body of an epizootic kills animals it affects so regularly that recovery is of very rare occurrence. The first animals affected in an outbreak, however, are sometimes only mildly ill and frequently recover. To me this fact strongly suggests that the hog cholera virus responsible for infecting the mild first cases originates in a reservoir host, other than swine, in which it has undergone some modification or attenuation. A single passage of the mild reservoir virus in swine appears to restore it to full pathogenicity, and it then progresses throughout a swine drove as the killer it is known typically to be. This hypothetical reservoir host for hog cholera virus has not yet been discovered and still presents an intriguing problem for study. It must exist, however, as no other hypothesis fits the known facts of the epidemiology of hog cholera. Certainly the epidemiological facts involving mild first cases are not consistent with the popularly held conception that hog cholera in a swine drove stems from established cases of the disease in neighboring droves.

RABBIT FIBROMATOSIS

Rabbit fibromatosis is a virus disease of cottontail rabbits. In a large number of naturally occurring cases that I have personally observed, the tumorous masses have been on one or more of the feet of the affected animal in all except one case. In the single exception the fibroma arose from the skin of a shoulder. Since it is known, from a large amount of experimental work, that fibromas occur only at sites at which virus is actually introduced, it follows that, under natural conditions, in cottontail rabbits, the feet constitute the portal of entry in the large majority of instances. It might be reasoned from this that the virus entered through abrasions on the feet. I personally doubt this explanation because the feet of the cottontail are well protected by a mass of thick, coarse hair, and almost any other part of the animal's body would be as subject to abrasions from thorns and other sharp objects as are the feet. I would rather interpret the almost specific localization of the tumors to the feet as indicating that the virus is transmitted by some intermediate host which inhabits the soil—perhaps of the woodchuck burrows which the cottontail frequents—and gains access to the feet of the rabbit by skin penetration. Several worm parasites of rabbits are known to penetrate skin in a manner analogous to that of the hookworm in man. The possibility is completely hypothetical and unproven, but to me it seems to constitute a definite clue pointing perhaps in a fruitful direction.

SALMON POISONING

The next example that I should like to cite is one of those diseases of unknown etiology. Salmon poisoning is an acute, highly fatal disease of dogs and other *Canidae* limited to that portion of Northwestern California, Western Oregon, and Southwestern Washington lying west of the Cascade Mountains. It is an old disease, having been recognized since the Pacific Northwest was first settled by white men and their dogs. Practical dog owners living along the streams and rivers of the area in which salmon poisoning prevails have long contended that the disease was a definite and distinct clinical entity which resulted when their dogs ate salmon or trout (1). It was not until Donham (2) in 1925 reported finding an intestinal fluke in dogs dying of the disease that any definite knowledge of the real cause was available. He found the encysted metacercariae of this fluke in both salmon and trout, produced the disease by feeding these metacercariae to dogs, and recovered the matured parasites from his experimentally fed animals. Donham believed that his experiments indicated this fluke to be the actual cause of salmon poisoning. It was named *Nanophyetus salmincola* by Chapin (3), who described it. Later it was shown that the snail host of the fluke was *Goniobasis plicifera* (4). This discovery explained the geographical distribution of the disease, as the snail in question has been collected only in those sections where salmon poisoning occurs. For about seven years Donham's fluke seemed to fill the role of the etiological agent in salmon poisoning satisfactorily. However, certain features of the disease were incompatible with the fluke theory of causation, and it was these that led to further work and a clearer understanding of the actual role played by the fluke. It was recognized by people working with the disease that it had many characteristics of an acute infection: the definite incubation period, the sudden onset, the severe systemic reaction, the rapid course, and the definite immunity in those few dogs which recovered. In crucial experiments published in 1932 (5) it was demonstrated that an infectious agent separable from the fluke was capable of producing the clinical picture of salmon poisoning. It was found that blood taken from dogs acutely ill following the ingestion of fluke-infested fish contained an agent that was transmissible serially to other dogs. Such blood, given either subcutaneously or intraperitoneally, caused a disease identical with that resulting from the ingestion of parasitized fish. The infectious agent could be passed successively from dog to dog by blood transfer, though in no case was it transmitted by contact. It was apparent from this work that the true cause of salmon poisoning was an infectious agent carried by the worm but separable from it. The exact nature of this agent remains unknown; it has thus far not been cultivated nor seen microscopically and would appear to be in the nature of a virus.

In salmon poisoning we thus have an infectious disease which under natural conditions exists entirely in what might be termed "first cases." Not being contagious, the disease never progresses beyond the initial fluke-transmitted case. However, since the causative agent is present in the blood stream, a set of conditions can be visualized in which, by the introduction of a bloodsucking vector into the cycle, the disease might be transformed into one which could progress widely throughout a dog population much as do some of the better-known insect-transmitted viruses among other hosts. If this hypothetical situation, that of transmission of salmon poisoning among dogs by an intermediate insect host, had existed at the time salmon poisoning was first subjected to experimental study, I should like to hazard the guess that we would not yet be aware of the fact that the first cases originated from an obscure fluke in a fish reservoir host. The clue indicating that a fluke in fish was involved as reservoir and intermediate host had to be furnished by circumstantial evidence that probably would have been overlooked had any direct dog-to-dog transmitting mechanism been operative.

BOVINE PSEUDORABIES

The next disease that I should like briefly to discuss from the standpoint of epidemiologic clues is bovine pseudorabies. This is an acute, highly fatal disease of cattle caused by the pseudorabies virus.

Throughout the Middle West, where it is most prevalent, the disease is known popularly as "mad itch" from its cardinal clinical feature, an extreme pruritis in which the animals mutilate an area of skin somewhere on their bodies by persistently licking and biting at it. Death always ensues, usually within thirty-six to forty-eight hours of the time the animal is first noticed to be affected. As a rule, only a small portion of a herd is involved, and it is not uncommon to have single cases observed in rather large groups of animals. Bovine pseudorabies never reaches epizootic proportions, and long periods of time may elapse between individual cases in a community. Many farms escape infection, even in areas where the disease is known to be enzootic. The disease has no recognized seasonal incidence.

The epidemiologic facts that I have just outlined suggest that pseudorabies is not contagious in cattle and that a secondary host of some sort must be responsible for its spread from animal to animal. In the early days, rats were suspected of being the intermediate host (6, 7, 8). The basis for this suspicion was the observation that not infrequently, on farms where pseudorabies was occurring in cattle, rats showing evidence of having died of an itching disease were sometimes found. In several instances, pseudorabies virus was actually demonstrated in the brains of these dead rats. Investigators who maintained that the rat might be the intermediate host responsible for the infection of cattle, however, never clearly visualized in just what manner rats might transmit the virus to cattle. Some suggested that it might be by biting. The weakness of this suggestion is that virus has never been detected in the mouths or saliva of infected rats.

In the first outbreak of bovine pseudorabies that I observed personally (9), no rats were found on the farm at the time that the disease was killing the cattle. The owner stated, however, that rats had been present earlier and that dead rats had been observed around the barn and barn lot as recently as one week before the occurrence of pseudorabies in the cattle. Consideration of this particular outbreak of pseudorabies made it apparent that the cattle had acquired their infection in the barn lot and furthermore emphasized the noncontagiousness of the disease in cattle. The group of cattle in which all of the cases occurred on this farm had been kept in the barn and barn lot until the first cases appeared (10). After this they were turned out to a near-by pasture during the daytime

THE SPREAD OF VIRUSES

with a large group of young steers and heifers, feeding with them and drinking from a common watering trough. No case of pseudorabies occurred among the steers and heifers, despite intimate contact with frank cases in the pasture. There were nine fatal cases of the disease, however, in the group of cattle that had been kept in the barn lot. It was apparent that the answer to the riddle of the epidemiology of pseudorabies lay right in this Iowa barn lot, and I am chagrined to have to say that I did not learn that answer from the clues furnished. I examined the barn lot carefully, and it seemed to present no features differing in any way from those of hundreds of other Midwestern farms. I was particularly interested in its livestock population, thinking of the possibility that some other host might be responsible for spreading the disease to cattle. There was a dog and there were several cats on the place. In addition, there were numerous chickens on free range with access to the barn lot, and in the barn lot itself were a fair number of swine. The dogs, cats, chickens, and swine all appeared healthy, and, on questioning the owner, I learned that no illness of any sort had been observed in any of them. The cattle had not been off the place and no new stock had been recently introduced. The only incriminating bit of evidence seemed to point to the former rat population of the farm. Since the rats had by then vanished they could not be investigated. I left the farm with the feeling that here was an instance in which the epidemiology of an isolated outbreak of disease might have been worked out had there been a more thorough understanding of the properties and behavior of the causative virus under experimental conditions.

The pseudorabies virus was intensively studied for the next several years, and from this work came an explanation of the epidemiology of the disease it causes in cattle. It was found that, although the pseudorabies virus caused a rapidly fatal itching disease when administered subcutaneously to cattle or any of the small laboratory animals, it induced only a mild and ill-defined transient illness when similarly administered to swine. Furthermore, pseudorabies in swine proved to be highly contagious, in contrast to its noncontagiousness in cattle and other experimental animals (10). Its mild but highly contagious character thus fitted it, potentially at least, as an ideal reservoir infection. It was found that it was transmitted from swine to swine by way of the nasal passages, and in some instances virus could be detected in or on the noses of infected swine for as long as ten days. Pseudorabies could be transmitted from swine to rabbits merely by bringing the noses of infected swine into contact with abraded areas of skin on rabbits. To one familiar with the behavior of swine when they are with cattle it seemed likely that a virus present in and on the nose of a hog could be readily transferred to the skin of a cow, because cattle lying about a barn lot in which hogs are also kept come frequently into contact with the hogs' noses.

With this lead as to the possible epidemiological mechanism involved in bovine pseudorabies, further natural outbreaks were studied on Iowa farms. It was noted that all cases occurred on farms where swine and cattle were kept together in the same enclosures. In two outbreaks—the only ones in which the matter was studied—pseudorabies virus-neutralizing antibodies found to be present in the sera of swine associated with the infected cattle indicated that the swine had undergone a previous infection with pseudorabies virus (10). A point of some interest was that no illness had been noted in these swine by their owners: that is, the porcine pseudorabies infections had been completely "silent." In the cattle on these farms, on the other hand, the disease progressed rapidly to a fatal end once they acquired a pseudorabies virus infection. The fact that pseudorabies virus-neutralizing antibodies were not present in the sera of any of the cattle surviving the outbreaks indicated that no subclinical bovine infections occurred and that all cattle in which virus infections were established died.

The evidence that I have presented, while admittedly circumstantial, indicates strongly that cattle become infected with pseudorabies virus by contact with infected swine. Pseudorabies in swine is a highly contagious disease and, judged on the basis of the presence of virus-neutralizing antibodies, is a widespread, though unrecognized, disease in Middle Western hogs—a silent epizootic (11). The presence of pseudorabies on a farm or in a community is recognized only when it escapes from a swine population and spreads to cattle. Usually this escape is limited and is reflected only in sporadic cases. Bovine pseudorabies, being not contagious, does not spread, and each case constitutes in reality a blind-alley infection. Were it not for its porcine intermediate and reservoir host to perpetuate it, pseudorabies

THE SPREAD OF VIRUSES

virus would die out and be forever lost in the first cow it killed. It is evident, I believe, that the apparent sporadicity of bovine pseudorabies is merely the epidemiological artifact resulting when a virus which induces a silent, though highly contagious, disease in one host spreads from that host to one in which it causes a recognizable, though noncontagious, ailment. I wonder how many other sporadic diseases represent similar epidemiological artifacts without the advantage, for purposes of study, of having a wide susceptible host spectrum, as does pseudorabies virus. It would be unexpected for nature to create a model for disease dissemination as intricate as that for pseudorabies and not to use it again.

SWINE INFLUENZA

The last disease that I should like to discuss from the standpoint of clues indicating the origin of virus responsible for its first cases, is swine influenza. Swine influenza may be defined as an acute, highly contagious, respiratory disease of hogs caused by *Hemophilus influenzae suis* and the swine influenza virus acting in concert. Its onset is sudden and the morbidity rate in an infected herd approximates 100 per cent.

Swine influenza epizootics have occurred in the Middle West each year since 1918. Characteristically they begin explosively late in October or early in November (12, 13). The build-up in cases is extremely rapid, and one gains the impression that the disease either spreads like wildfire or has arisen at many foci simultaneously. The disease, if it is actually disseminated from farm to farm, gets spread about in miraculously rapid fashion—in fact, so rapidly that the theory of spread from farm to farm by actual contact is an almost unbelievable hypothesis. The pattern of apparent dissemination of swine influenza among farms is very reminiscent of that seen among army camps and civilian communities at the outset of the 1918 human pandemic. After the initial widespread outbreak, fresh swine droves become infected in smaller and smaller numbers until by late December, as a rule, the epizootic appears to have run its course, and swine influenza disappears as a farm infection until the following October or November. The bacterial component of the etiological complex, *H. influenzae suis*, can persist indefinitely in the upper respiratory tracts of some recovered swine. However, similar persistence of the virus cannot be demonstrated.

The whereabouts of the swine influenza virus during interepizootic periods and the origin of that infecting the first cases in a succeeding epizootic were for many years unsuspected. While clues indicating that it must persist right on the affected farms from year to year were numerous, they were not explicit enough to enable one to determine just which of the numerous possibilities might be most profitable for exhaustive study. Among those that I considered most likely, and which I have from time to time tried to incriminate, were virus carriers among the pigs themselves, migrating birds, the small rodents which move from the fields to the barns and barn lots each autumn, and even the corn which is husked and brought to the barn lot at about the beginning of the influenza season. None of these clues proved to be the right one, and it was an entirely accidental observation that finally settled the issue. The observation was made in two stages: First, it was found that swine could be carriers of masked swine influenza virus which by certain manipulations could be provoked to infectivity (14). Secondly, it was found that swine acquired these masked swine influenza virus infections through an intermediate host, the swine lungworm (15). I regret to say that three years were required to work from the first to the second stage, and even then a great deal of good luck was involved.

The intermediate host system whereby swine influenza virus from one epizootic is preserved to infect the first cases of a succeeding epizootic is not a simple one. The swine lungworm is the actual reservoir and intermediate host of the virus. However, the lungworm has an intermediate host of its own, the common earthworm, and must spend three of its developmental stages in its earthworm intermediate host before it can parasitize swine (16, 17). Swine acquire their lungworms by eating earthworms (gotten by rooting in the soil) infested with third-stage lungworm larvae. If these lungworm larvae were hatched from eggs laid by an adult lungworm while she was infesting the lung of a pig with influenza they will be carriers of masked influenza virus. The pig acquiring the larvae will then become infected with masked virus when the larvae migrate to its respiratory tract. The term "masked" is applied to virus in its lung-

THE SPREAD OF VIRUSES

worm intermediate host to indicate that it is present there in an occult and not directly detectable form. Swine infested with lungworm carriers of this masked swine influenza virus remain normal to all appearances, and there is no way of detecting directly that they are actually carrying swine influenza virus. However, such swine are in a very precarious situation as far as their eventual well-being is concerned, because all that is required to bring them down with a severe, or perhaps even fatal, attack of swine influenza is the application of some stimulus, of itself relatively harmless. Several such provocative stimuli have been used, but the one that has proved most regularly effective consists in the administration of multiple intramuscular injections of the bacterium *H. influenza suis*. Under natural conditions on the farm the provocative stimulus is probably meteorological in character, being in some way associated with the onset of wet, cold, inclement weather.

The intermediate host mechanism that I have briefly outlined adequately accounts for the perpetuation of swine influenza. It has been found that virus can persist for at least as long as thirty-two months in third-stage lungworm larvae in their earthworm intermediate hosts, and for at least an additional three months in association with adult lungworms in the swine respiratory tract (18). This constitutes a total elapsed time—between the case of swine influenza originally supplying the virus and the hog eventually becoming infected with it—of almost three years, roughly three times the period which must be accounted for to explain the survival of the virus from one epizootic to the next.

There is evidence from some field work on the subject that the incidence of swine infected with masked virus may be quite high (19). This would suggest that the apparent paradox of swine influenza spreading throughout a drove and from farm to farm faster, we realize, than it can on the basis of any known incubation period may not be a paradox at all. The field evidence indicates that the virus is probably widely seeded before the outbreak and is merely provoked almost simultaneously in large geographical areas by a common stimulus. The great rapidity of spread may, therefore, be more apparent than real. I do not mean to imply that swine influenza does not ordinarily behave like a typical contagious disease in spreading from sick to well animals. I am certain that it does; in the laboratory under experimental conditions, it can be shown to be regularly and highly contagious. The point that I should like to emphasize, however, is that in swine influenza the number of first cases responsible for initiating an epizootic may be larger than in most contagious diseases and that this may account for the thoroughness with which it involves an entire swine population.

Now to get back to this question of clues indicating the origin of the virus responsible for first cases of swine influenza. I think that it was very evident, from consideration of the epidemiology of individual outbreaks, that the virus source had to be on the involved farm itself. However, I must admit that there was little to suggest searching underground for it.

This concludes what I have to say about the spread of viruses from infected to susceptible hosts. I have tried to indicate, by the examples I have cited, the devious means by which certain viruses are perpetuated in nature and by which they get from the infected hosts of one outbreak of disease to the susceptible hosts of the next. I have also tried to point out that consideration of the natural history of an outbreak of disease may yield a clue as to the origin of the virus responsible for it. Greenwood, in one of his Herter Lectures (20), phrased the thought a little more subtly when he stated: "Although the book of nature and human fate contains the answers to all our epidemiological questions, we do not know enough of the grammar of the language in which it is written to understand these answers." A plea that I should like to add to Greenwood's statement is that in trying to solve the problems of the epidemiology of the virus diseases we concentrate as much on our grammar as on our mathematics.

REFERENCES

1. Simms, B. T., C. R. Donham, and J. N. Shaw, Salmon poisoning, *J. Am. Vet. Med. Assn.*, 1931, 78:181.
2. Donham, C. R., So-called salmon poisoning of dogs, *J. Am. Vet. Med. Assn.*, 1925, 66:637.
3. Chapin, E. A., A new genus and species of trematode, the probable cause of salmon poisoning in dogs, *No. Am. Vet.*, 1926, 7:36.
4. Donham, C. R., B. T. Simms, and J. N. Shaw, *Salmon Poisoning in Dogs* (Motion picture film, Oregon State Agr. Coll., 1927).
5. Simms, B. T., A. M. McCapes, and O. H. Muth, Salmon poisoning:

Transmission and immunization experiments, *J. Am. Vet. Med. Assn.*, 1932, 81:26.

6. Schmiedhoffer, J., Beitrage zur Pathologie der Infektiösen Bulbärparalyse (Aujeszkyschen Krankheit), *Ztschr. Infektionskrankh. Haustiere*, 1910, 8:383.
7. Hutyra, F., Beitrage zur Ätiologie der Infektiösen Bulbärparalyse, *Berl. tierärztl. Wchnschr.* 1910, 26:149.
8. Burggraaf, A., and L. F. D. E. Lourens, Infectieuse Bulbair–Paralyse (Ziekte van Aujeszky), *Tijdschr. Diergeneesk.*, 1932, 59:981.
9. Shope, R. E., An experimental study of "mad itch" with especial reference to its relationship to pseudorabies, *J. Exp. Med.*, 1931, 54:233.
10. Shope, R. E., Experiments on the epidemiology of pseudorabies I. Mode of transmission of the disease in swine and their possible role in its spread to cattle, *J. Exp. Med.*, 1935, 62:85.
11. Shope, R. E., Experiments on the epidemiology of pseudorabies, II: Prevalence of the disease among Middle Western swine and the possible role of rats in herd-to-herd infections, *J. Exp. Med.*, 1935, 62:101.
12. Dorset, M. C., C. N. McBryde, and W. B. Niles, Remarks on "hog flu," *J. Am. Vet. Med. Assn.*, 1922, 62:162.
13. McBryde, C. N., Some observations on "hog flu" and its seasonal prevalence in Iowa, *J. Am. Vet. Med. Assn.*, 1927, 71:368.
14. Shope, R. E., The swine lungworm as a reservoir and intermediate host for swine influenza virus; I: The presence of swine influenza virus in healthy and susceptible pigs, *J. Exp. Med.*, 1941, 74:41.
15. Shope, R. E., The swine lungworm as a reservoir and intermediate host for swine influenza virus, II: The transmission of swine influenza virus by the swine lungworm, *J. Exp. Med.*, 1941, 74:49.
16. Hobmaier, A., and M. Hobmaier, Die Entwicklung der Larve des Lungenwurmes *Metastrongylus elongatus* (*Strongylus paradoxus*) des Schweines und ihr Invasionsweg, sowie Zorläufige Mitteilung über die Entwicklung von *Choerostrongylus brevivaginatus*, *Münch. tierärztl. Wchnschr.*, 1929, 80:365. Biologie von *Choerostrongylus* (*Metastrongylus*) *pudendotectus* (*brevivaginatus*) aus der Lunge des Schweines, guglelch eine Vorläufige Mitteilung über die Entwicklung der Gruppe Synthetocaulus unserer Haustiere, *Münch. tierärztl. Wchnschr*, 1929, 80:433.
17. Schwartz, B., and J. E. Alicata, The development of Metastrongylus elongatus in their intermediate hosts (abstract), *J. Parasitol.*, 1929, 16:105. Concerning the life history of lungworms of swine, *J. Parasitol.*, 1931, 18:21. *Life history of lungworms parasitic in swine*, U. S. Dept. Agric. Tech. Bull. 456, 1934.
18. Shope, R. E., The swine lungworm as a reservoir and intermediate host for swine influenza virus, III: Factors influencing transmission of the virus and the provocation of influenza, *J. Exp. Med.*, 1943, 77:111.
19. Shope, R. E., The swine lungworm as a reservoir and intermediate host

for swine influenza virus, IV: The demonstration of masked swine influenza virus in lungworm larvae and swine under natural conditions, *J. Exp. Med.*, 1943, 77:127.
20. Greenwood, M., *Epidemiology Historical and Experimental* (The Herter Lectures for 1931, Baltimore, 1932).

Chapter 3

THE CULTURE AND EFFECTS OF VIRUSES IN CHICK EMBRYO CELLS

By G. John Buddingh, *Louisiana State University School of Medicine*

An abiding interest in the pathology and pathogenesis of viral infections prompted Goodpasture and his associates to an important series of experimental investigations. Motivated by the hypothesis of the exclusive multiplication within living cells, these studies emphasized the concept of cytotropism as basic to an understanding of the behavior and nature of viruses. The demonstration of the intracellular presence of fowl-pox virus and its relation to the specific cellular inclusion of this disease was directly antecedent to a resort to the use of the developing chick embryo for the study of the cytology and pathogenesis of viral infections (1).

If the concept of cytotropism as it relates to the characteristic adaptation of viruses to host cells is to develop a more precise and fundamental distinction, it must be elaborated to embrace a characterization of those metabolic processes which specifically identify susceptible cells. Certain observations have been made in the course of various studies on the culture of viruses and on the pathogenesis of viral infections of the chick embryo which, if further explored, may prove of significance in this direction.

Empirical observations, the immediate exigencies of the moment with its practical demand for viruses in quantity, and the necessity for technical simplicity have to a great extent determined the stage of embryonic development and the route of inoculation best suited for the propagation of different viruses. Very few data are available to provide a reasonable explanation why, for example, the rickettsiae multiply best in the yolk sac of six-to eight-day embryos or why equine encephalomyelitis virus is cultured in greatest quantity in the tissues of seven- to nine-day embryos, influenza virus, following introduction into the allantoic cavity of ten- to eleven-day embryos, or vaccinia, in the chorio-allantois of twelve- to fourteen-day embryos.

The embryonated hen's egg is not just a convenient receptacle in which viruses and other infectious agents find suitable conditions for their multiplication. Under the proper conditions of incubation the fertile egg proceeds at a furious rate. From hour to hour, day to day, the successive steps of development and differentiation which complete the hatched chick within 21 days confront us with a series of biochemical and biophysical situations to which viruses are variously adapted.

During a definite stage of development, particularly from the twelfth through the fifteenth day of incubation, infection of the embryo with a wide variety of viruses is most likely to reproduce, to a significant degree of similarity, those cellular and inflammatory reactions characteristically observed in the naturally susceptible host in the post-embryonic stage. Thus infection of the twelve-day chorio-allantois with fowl-pox virus, perhaps more than any other, simulates the natural lesions of the disease. The characteristic predilection of the virus for epithelial cells is strikingly illustrated. The hypertrophy and hyperplasia, especially of the ectodermal epithelium and to a lesser degree of the endodermal epithelium, and the occurrence within these cells of the pathognomonic Bollinger bodies are typical of this infection. Although the virus can be demonstrated in the bloodstream, generalization of the infection to the embryo does not seem to occur by this route (2).

Vaccinia virus is readily propagated in the chorio-allantois of twelve- to fifteen-day embryos. Grossly characteristic pock-like eruptions develop within forty-eight to seventy-two hours (3). Elementary bodies in great abundance can be demonstrated in properly stained smears made from these lesions. The cytology of the reaction to vaccinal infection of the membrane reveals many of the features typical of the lesion in the natural disease. The predominantly selective affinity of this virus for epithelial cells asserts itself. The immediate response of the ectodermal epithelium to invasion by the virus is that of hypertrophy and hyperplasia in the form of focal proliferations. Many of the cells in such foci contain characteristic cytoplasmic inclusions. The virus multiplies rapidly within them and their destruction is quickly effected. Widespread ulceration of the ectodermal epithelium is typical of membrane infection with vaccinia.

Most dermal strains of vaccinia virus which are generally used in this country for smallpox vaccination have a more or less marked capacity for invading the fibroblasts and endothelial cells of the mesoderm and the endodermal cells of the chorio-allantois. Upon continued serial passage in the membrane, the capacity of the virus for infecting mesodermal cells gradually disappears. This enhanced epidermotropism is reflected in the nature of the reaction produced by embryo-adapted vaccinia in the rabbit skin. A more superficial and mild reaction in which the evolution of the lesion is accelerated, as compared with infection produced by calf-propagated virus, develops. This modification apparently does not affect the antigenic qualities of the virus (4).

This enhancement of a more restricted epidermotropism may perhaps be due to a selective process by which the major part of a virus population in which affinity for ectodermal epithelial cells is most pronounced is retained. while that part with mesothelial and endodermal affinities fails to survive. The evidence at present available does not permit definite conclusions regarding this possibility. It is of great interest that generalization of the infection to the embryo by way of the blood stream from the chorio-allantoic lesion takes place with great regularity with these membrane adapted strains (5). Transported to the embryo. the same virus which in the membrane restricts its activity to ectodermal epithelium in duces infection of the cells of various organs and tissues. Focal lesions in which many cells contain typical inclusions can be found in the liver, myocardium, striated muscle, meninges, and other tissues of endodermal and mesodermal origin. In the later stages of the generalized infection pock-like eruptions of the skin of the embryo develop. Cytologically these lesions are astoundingly similar to those of the natural disease.

This striking transgression of the bounds of a well-established epidermotropism suggests that at this stage of embryonic development the cells of endodermal and mesodermal origin still maintain a substrate of metabolic processes which include reaction systems essential to the support of the virus. These reaction systems, whatever they may be, are perhaps more dominant or accessible to the virus in epithelial cells, and eventually may be found to characterize them as such. The mesodermal and endodermal cells of the chorio-allantois beyond the eleven-day stage very likely carry on physiological functions in which the metabolic activities to which a strict epidermotrop is adapted are suppressed or have disappeared.

This state of affairs is even more apparent when vaccinia virus is introduced into the amniotic sac of eight- or nine-day-old embryos. Under these circumstances the virus proliferates so rapidly that the embryo dies within twenty-four to thirty-six hours. The infectivity titer of the amniotic fluid at this period is comparable to that obtained from forty-eight- to seventy-two hour membranal infections of twelve-day embryos. The entire embryo can be used as a good source of virus. No grossly visible lesions other than scattered subcutaneous hemorrhages develop. Microscopic study reveals no proliferative lesions of the embryonic epidermis, nor are typical intracytoplasmic inclusions found. Superficial epithelial necrosis is evident but there is no true ulceration. Cellular multiplication at this stage is so rapid that parasitized cells are replaced as soon as they are destroyed. The rate of virus proliferation seemingly keeps pace with the rate of multiplication of the susceptible cells (6).

In this instance the multiplication of virus is conditioned not primarily by a specific cell type but more than likely by the nature and rate of the metabolic processes which characterize embryonic development at this stage. Thus equine encephalomyelitis virus multiplies with exceeding rapidity in seven- or eight-day embryos. The Eastern and Western strains of this agent have a typical predilection for the central nervous system of the horse and man. In the developing embryo no such strict cytotropism apparently is maintained. Although it is not conclusively demonstrated, this infectious agent seems to exert a general assault on all the cells and tissues of the embryo (7). Observations on the rate of multiplication of this virus have been made only on ten-day embryos, but it is evident from Bang's studies that as embryonic development advances the rate of multiplication of the virus, as judged from mortality rates, gradually diminishes (7).

A most significant and penetrating analysis of these factors has been presented by Crawley (8). Comparison of the LD 50 mortality end points of embryos inoculated by the chorio-allantoic route with equine encephalomyelitis virus indicates the marked susceptibility of eight-day-old embryos and the gradual daily decrease in susceptibility with advancing development through fifteen days of incubation. Remarkably, eight-day embryos with a high degree of susceptibility to chorio-allantoic inoculation with the virus show a degree of insusceptibility following yolk-sac inoculation comparable to 15-day embryos infected by the membranal route. Conversely, fifteen-day embryos inoculated by way of the yolk sac exhibit a degree of susceptibility encountered in eight-day embryos inoculated by the membranal route. An explanation of this seeming paradox is presented by proposing that the increasing resistance to infection by the chorio-allantoic route may be attributed to physiological aging and lack of developing young cells in the chorio-allantois. On the other hand, the gradual increase in susceptibility to yolk-sac inoculation in older embryos is brought about by increased physiological function and an increase in the number of columnar cells of the yolk-sac membrane (8). These important observations imply a shift from one locality to another in the embryonated egg of as yet uncharacterized metabolic activities which are essential for the efficient multiplication of the virus.

A variety of response to infection is also observed with the virus of herpes simplex in the chick embryo at successive stages of development. This agent is readily propagated in the chorio-allantois (9). Anderson (10) has made a study of the pathogenesis of this experimental infection by a cytological analysis of the nature and distribution of the lesions following chorio-allantoic and intra-amniotic inoculation of the virus in embryos at various stages of development. Especially during the twelfth to the fifteenth day of incubation, infection of the chorio-allantois with herpes virus reproduces the basic cytological features of dermal lesion of the natural disease. There is an early proliferative response of ectodermal epithelium during which the typical intranuclear inclusions are readily detected in the parasitized cells. Destruction of the invaded cells progresses rapidly, and widespread necrosis of ectodermal epithelium is encountered within forty-eight to seventy-two hours. In the later stages of infection parasitization of mesodermal cells of the membrane is evidenced by the presence of intranuclear inclusions in fibroblasts and endothelial cells. The studies of Shaffer and Enders (11) seem to indicate a greater degree of susceptibility of the fifteen-day chorio-allantois as compared with that of twelve- to thirteen-day incubation. Anderson's observations suggest a definite modification in response to infection in the chorio-allantois of embryos inoculated on the sixteenth day of incubation. She states: "The reaction to infection was purely a proliferative one, limited to the ectodermal epithelium without necrosis or spread of the infection to the underlying mesoderm." This is in some respects analogous to the observations mentioned above regarding the reaction to infection with chick embryo adapted vaccinia virus in the twelve-day-old chorio-allantois. By the seventeenth day the membranal mesodermal cells no longer carry on those metabolic activities possessed on the twelfth day which support the multiplication of herpes simplex. The ectodermal epithelium, however, apparently retains a pattern of biochemical activities which are essential to this virus.

Generalization of herpetic infection by way of the blood stream to the embryo regularly occurs following chorio-allantoic inoculation of twelve- or thirteen-day embryos. Invasion of the brain occurred only during the first membranal passages of the highly neurotropic HF strain of the virus. Elsewhere metastatic lesions, specifically identified by the presence of typical intranuclear inclusions, develop in practically all tissues and organs of the embryo. With adaptation to the embryonic host the virus loses its capacity to infect nervous tissue when disseminated from the membrane by way of the blood stream, and the predilection for tissue cells of mesodermal origin becomes accentuated (10).

Membrane-adapted virus introduced directly into the embryo brain was found to incite a typical herpetic encephalitis. This peculiar modification of a strain of herpes virus with high initial neurotropic potentialities was further indicated by the fact that after twenty membranal passages it was no longer possible to induce herpetic encephalitis in rabbits after corneal inoculation. Direct intracerebral injection, however, produced a typical encephalitis.

The epidermal predilection of herpes virus is especially well demonstrated after intra-amniotic inoculation. Typical vesicular lesions of the skin and the mucous membranes of the pharynx, and a widespread involvement of the amniotic cells develop. When the virus is introduced subcutaneously in thirteen-day ambryos typical lesions develop at the site of inoculation. In one embryo thus treated, an ascending myelitis with involvement of the spinal cord at the level of inoculation was observed (10).

These observations on herpetic infection emphasize that at least up to the sixteenth day of incubation a great variety, and perhaps all, of the cells of the embryo share in a biological substrate to which herpes virus is adapted. The essential cytotropism of the virus is known to be maintained, since cytological evidence of the intracellular presence of the virus in all foci of infection is readily obtained. However, in the embryo the virus is not restricted to the neurotropism and epidermotropism exhibited in other experimental and natural hosts in post embryonic life. In the later stages of embryonic development, at least in so far as observations on the chorio-allantois are concerned, the metabolic and other biological substrates which eventually characterize epithelial cells are established and distinguish them from mesodermal cells. Beyond the sixteenth day of incubation to the nineteenth day apparently only ectodermal epithelium supports the multiplication of the virus of herpes simplex.

In this instance it seems unlikely that propagation in the embryo exerts a selective activity upon such constituents of the original virus moiety which favors the survival of or enhances a particular tropism as it might relate to specific cell types. After long-continued passage in the chorio-allantois the virus, upon intra-amniotic inoculation, readily thrives in the epithelium of the skin. Upon intracerebral inoculation into the embryo or into rabbits it has lost little, if any, of its capacity to parasitize nervous tissues.

Although beyond the province of this discussion, it must be emphasized that propagation in the embryo is not without profound effect on viruses. Continued serial passage frequently results in increased adaptation and heightened virulence for the embryo. These modifications in many instances have been found to be reflected in diminished virulence and pathogenicity for susceptible experimental animals or the natural host.

For several of the viruses and rickettsiae which have been successfully adapted to embryo culture for vaccine purposes alterations in antigenic properties have not occurred to such an extent as to be of practical import. Yet the evidence available affords no certainty that the methods thus far found most suitable for the rapid and facile collection of viruses in quantity favor those conditions which will best maintain their original antigenic qualities.

Since William Harvey's day the embryologists and many other investigators have brought to light a great body of data and much knowledge regarding the chemical and physiological reactions which take place in the avian egg throughout all of its stages of development. Reference to such comprehensive compilations as Needham's *Chemical Embryology* (12) will reveal the extent of the information which is available regarding the chick embryo. There has been up to present time relatively little opportunity to relate observations on the culture of viruses and their effect on the embryo cells to these more fundamental efforts concerned with an elucidation of embryonic metabolism and physiology. At the moment, it is in no way proposed to discuss this field of knowledge authoritatively or with adequate understanding.

During the first seven or eight days of development the chick embryo cells in many respects resemble rapidly growing cultures of bacteria in that they show a marked inefficiency in the utilization of energy. The metabolic processes from which the energy sources are derived consist mainly of the combustion of carbohydrates—glucose derived from the albumin. During this first trimester cellular multiplication proceeds at its most rapid rate. The general metabolism is maintained at its highest peak of activity. In all probability all of the embryonic cells are characterized by metabolic process of the type in which glucose serves as the chief energy source. These processes are biologically less complicated and typical of more simple forms of life.

This feature of embryonic cellular metabolism perhaps indicates that during the first trimester of development certain metabolic common denominators are shared by all the embryonic cells. It may prove to be the key to their almost uniform susceptibility to infection with most, if not all, human and animal viruses. As was already indicated, the rapid rate of virus proliferation during this stage is perhaps determined by the equally rapid rate of cellular multiplication. Several analogies to phenomena observed with bacteriophages are evident under these circumstances.

It has not yet been determined if there exists in the very early hours or first one or two days of this first trimester a stage in which embryonic cells are insusceptible to viral infections. If such a period does exist there may be opportunity for determining what metabolic and other biological factors are fundamentally essential for viruses.

If, on the other hand, the earliest cells of the embryo are susceptible the behavior of viruses under these circumstances might prove highly illuminating.

About the tenth day of incubation the general metabolism and growth rate of the embryo undergo a marked and continuous relative retardation. Beginning about the ninth day the combustion of protein rather than of carbohydrates serves as a source of energy, which from this time onward is utilized with increasing efficiency. During this second trimester protein synthesis and breakdown predominantly characterize the cellular activities. Organization and differentiation of organs and tissues in respect to their morphology become more and more definitive.

It is obvious that during this second trimester of embryonic development viruses, as well as other infectious agents, are confronted with a biological substrate far different from that present during the first trimester. During the tenth to the twelfth day of incubation there very likely is a persistence in many cell types of some of the biological activities characteristic of the first trimester. It is at this stage especially that viruses, which exhibit a more selective cellular affinity in the more mature host, show a rather wide range of cellular adaptation. The formation of typical virus inclusions during this period may be due to a more definite and characteristic construction of the protein constituents of the susceptible cells.

With the more efficient utilization of energy and the accentuation of metabolic processes concerned with protein synthesis the reactions to viral infections more nearly approach those observed in the natural disease. The reduced rate of cellular multiplication quite likely induces a retardation in the rate of virus multiplication. Proliferative responses of typical cell types are at this time characteristically observed. It may be that as a result of a virus acting upon or in a substrate composed of more specifically defined proteins, reaction products develop which specifically stimulate proliferation of immediately surrounding cells.

Inflammatory reactions secondary to cellular destruction are characteristically observed during this stage. Before this it is possible that leucocytes and other cells which compose the inflammatory exudate have not sufficiently matured. It is, however, just as likely that the biochemical stimuli necessary for the mobilization of the inflammatory exudate can be derived only from parasitized cells in which the protein constituents have acquired a more characteristic composition.

As the fifteenth day of incubation, or the third trimester of development, approaches, cellular differentiation has reached a stage in which the specific metabolic activities and physiological functions which eventually characterize cells are to a large extent confined to each type. It has been noted that at this stage viruses are much more likely to exhibit specific cellular affinities than in younger embryonic cells. For viruses to which the hatched chick is insusceptible, species-specific characteristics begin to influence cellular susceptibilities at this time.

During the third trimester of embryonic development profound metabolic changes again take place. Preparations in anticipation of hatching are made in that the storage of energy in the form of fat derived from the yolk sac takes place. Fats, which constitute the most efficient biological source of energy, are mobilized and transported to the embryo. The cells of the yolk-sac membrane, which until then have been relatively quiescent, increase in size and number and assume a high degree of metabolic activity.

As was noted above, at this stage the embryo markedly increases in susceptibility to yolk-sac inoculation with encephalomyelitis virus. The accelerated metabolism involved to mobilizing fat by the yolk-sac cells provides the substrate which supports the proliferation of encephalomyelitis virus, rather than any type-specific quality of these cells as such.

The relative metabolic inactivity of yolk-sac cells during the first trimester is perhaps the main factor which favors the culture of rickettsiae. In their natural arachnid hosts the rickettsiae enjoy an environment in which metabolic activities very likely proceed at a more leisurely pace.

This much too brief outline should serve to emphasize the great range of potentialities of the chick embryo for the study of the relationship of viral agents to susceptible cells. The basic concept of cytotropism as it applies to the behavior of viruses is supported in all its implications by the phenomena observed in viral infections of the embryo. From no instance can it be concluded that viruses proliferate outside of or in the absence of living cells. There is an orderly progression of the embryonic metabolic activities from reaction patterns which characterize more simple bacterial cells in cultures to the highly complex activities of the specialized, organized, and differentiated cells of specific organs and tissues. Investigations toward relating the effects of viral agents on susceptible cells to facts already available regarding some of the basic manifestations of embryonic metabolism would well serve to elaborate the concept of cytotropism toward a more precise and fundamental distinction.

The necessity for adequate and critical cytological analyses of the processes involved in the pathogenesis of virus infections under the various distinct conditions presented at definite stages of embryonic development cannot be overemphasized. Progress in this direction will depend on a more intimate cooperative effort of virologists with those who have specialized in embryological morphology, physiology, and biochemistry.

The point of departure which has directed this discussion is not in any sense original. Final quotations from William Harvey's *De Generatione Animalibum* (13), published in 1651, should deprive it of any such pretension. "For while the foetus is yet feeble, Nature hath provided it with a milder diet and solider meats for its stronger capacity, and when it is now hearty enough, and can away with coarser cates, it is served with commons answerable to it." "About the fourth day the egg beginneth to step from the life of a plant to that of animal." "From that to the tenth it enjoys a sensitive and moving soul as animals do, and after that, it is completed by degrees and being adorned with Plumes, Bill, Clawes and other furniture, it hastens to get out."

REFERENCES

1. Goodpasture, E. W., The cell-parasite relationship in bacterial and virus infection. Alvarenga Prize Lecture. *Trans. & Studies Coll. Phys., Philadelphia*, 1941, 9:11.
2. Woodruff, A. M., and E. W. Goodpasture, The susceptibility of the chorio-allantoic membrane of chick embryos to infection with fowl-pox virus, *Am. J. Path.*, 1931, 7:209.
3. Goodpasture, E. W., A. M. Woodruff, and G. J. Buddingh, The cultivation of vaccinia and other viruses in the chorio-allantoic membrane of chick embryos, *Science*, 1931, 74:371.
4. Buddingh, G. J., The pathogenic and antigenic properties of dermal vaccinia virus propagated in the chorio-allantois of chick embryos, *Am. J. Hyg.*, 1943, 38:310.

5. Buddingh, G. J., A study of generalized infection of the chick embryo, *J. Exp. Med.*, 1936, 63:227.
6. Buddingh, G. J., Unpublished observations.
7. Bang, F., The course of experimental infection of the chick embryo with the virus of equine encephalomyelitis, *J. Exp. Med.*, 1943, 77:337.
8. Crawley, J. F., Statistical analysis of the factors affecting the susceptibility of chick embryos to eastern equine encephalomyelitis virus, *J. Immunol.*, 1948, 59:83.
9. Dawson, J. R., Herpetic infection of the chorio-allantoic membrane of chick embryos, *Am. J. Path.*, 1933, 9:1.
10. Anderson, K., Pathogenesis of herpes simplex virus infection of the chick embryo, *Am. J. Path.*, 1940, 16:137.
11. Shaffer, M. F., and J. F. Enders, Quantitative studies on the infectivity of the virus of herpes simplex for the chorio-allantoic membrane of the chick embryo, together with observations on the inactivation of the virus by its specific antiserum, *J. Immunol.*, 1939, 37:383.
12. Needham, J., *Chemical Embryology*, Vols. I, II, III, (New York, 1931).
13. Quoted from J. Needham, *Chemical Embryology*, Vol. I (New York, 1931).

Chapter 4

THE RELATIONSHIPS OF VIRUSES AND CELLS, WITH PARTICULAR REFERENCE TO THE INTERFERENCE PHENOMENON

By GILBERT DALLDORF, *Division of Laboratories and Research, New York State Department of Health*

OF ALL KNOWN host-parasite relationships, that between virus and cell is the most intimate. We might say that the cell completes the virus and gives it life. The two may form an "enduring partnership," as Doctor Kidd (1) described the union of papilloma virus and carcinoma cells, or an unholy alliance which is quickly followed by death. In both, the association is profound. We shall need to know much more about the structure and activities of viruses and cells before that relationship becomes clear.

Meanwhile, as often happens in biology, we have learned several things through indirection which help us to understand. We have discovered some of the factors which influence the union of the two. It seems to me that these might be appropriately considered at this time, because they supplement by a discussion of its final stages what Doctor Shope has said of the transmission of infection and because they suggest additional means by which viral diseases may some day be controlled.

The union of virus and cell is usually described as an adsorption, but the record shows that an irreversible reaction occurs between the two which gives adsorption of virus a very special meaning. The union is quick and final. Rous and his colleagues (2) mixed isolated cells with vaccinia and fibroma viruses and found they combined so quickly it was impossible to mix and separate. Within the briefest interval they could test, union was sufficiently complete to be no longer influenced by immune serum. It is fortunate for us that mechanisms exist which may prevent such rapid and irrevocable infection.

A virus may reach a susceptible host but never come in contact with the susceptible cells and therefore fail to infect. Humoral antibodies may intervene. Andrewes (3) showed that antiserum injected into the skin a few minutes before the inoculation of vaccinia virus prevented infection. Five minutes after inoculation it did not—further evidence of the rapidity of the union of the two. Chemical reagents, such as zinc sulfate and picric acid and alum, may prevent the invasion of the olfactory nerves by poliomyelitis virus (4). Exudative inflammation of the upper respiratory mucosa protected mice from St. Louis encephalitis virus instilled into their nares. Armstrong (5) found that mice first infected with a mixture of bacteria had double the survival rate of the noninfected ones. He thought the protection was "the result of a nonspecific type of local stimulation [which is] accompanied by an outpouring of leucocytes." A heavy exudate might conceivably prevent contact of virus with cells or a discharge purge the nares of an inoculum. But since bacterial filtrates and killed cultures were also effective, one is tempted to look further, and most workers today would suspect that his cultures contained an inhibitory substance.

A variety of substances is now known to inhibit the union of viruses and cells. Information has come from two sources: from the chemists who have sought to apply to this problem what has been learned from the chemotherapy of bacterial diseases and nutrition, and from those biologists who have analyzed the phenomenon by which certain viruses cause red blood cells to agglutinate. The evidence indicates that this useful and simple experiment which Hirst (6) discovered in 1942 is a model of virus infection, for what happens in the test tube and is revealed by hemagglutination, frequently happens *in vivo*, as well.

The essentials of the reaction are that virus first combines with the red blood cells, which thereupon agglutinate, and later is eluted, leaving the cells unable to further adsorb virus. Hirst postulated that the virus possesses an enzyme which destroys the cell's receptors and suggested that certain substances which prevent hemagglutination do so by substituting for the cell receptors. By combining with the virus, they block its union with the cell. The recent report by Lanni and Beard (7) of the dynamics of the reaction supports this theory. Hirst (8) further found that the cell receptor function and the inhibitory effect of normal serum were similar in several properties. Both were destroyed by sodium periodate and trypsin, as well as by influenza virus. These chemical considerations led to the idea that carbohydrate-protein complexes, such as mucin, play a role in the inhibition phenomenon, and a variety of mucins from different sources have been tested and some have been shown to be inhibitory. Burnet (9) concludes that the cell receptor is a mucin which is attacked by an appropriate enzyme from the surface of the influenza virus. Conversely, an insusceptible cell would be one without an appropriate mucin.

A modification of Hirst's explanation is proposed by Australian workers (9) to cover their observations of the behavior of periodate-treated cells and the role of an enzyme of *V. cholerae*. The treated cells adsorb virus but no longer elute it. Furthermore, such cells fail to fix the bacterial enzyme which normally destroys red cell receptors; and the enzyme cannot prevent treated cells from taking up virus nor elute adsorbed virus. *Part* of the receptor function has been destroyed. Anderson (10) therefore suggests that a larger cell structure is involved in the adsorption of virus than is destroyed by the virus enzyme. Only those parts—certain groupings in the receptor area—which are destroyed are responsible for elution, and it is only these which react with periodate. The modified theory, he points out, fits Burnet's discovery (11) of a gradient relationship between viruses as regards adsorption, since it allows for several successive combinations, each destructive only of the particular groupings which react specifically with an individual virus.

Other workers also have identified inhibitors with cell receptors. Bovarnick and de Burgh (12, 13) isolated from red cell stroma by ether extraction an inhibitor more active than others, which they consider to be receptor substance. The fraction contains 50-percent carbohydrate. Extracts of various human organs having an inhibitory effect upon hemagglutination have also been identified with cell receptor substance by Friedewald and his colleagues (14).

Inhibitory phenomena of a different kind have been discovered by Ginsberg, Goebel, and Horsfall (15). It had first been noted by Horsfall and McCarty (16) that certain polysaccharides modify the course of infection of mice with the pneumonia virus. Later it was learned that the capsular polysaccharide of Friedlander's bacillus inhibits the growth of mumps virus in fertile eggs. Here the inhibitor does not block the union of virus and cell but modifies the cell's metabolism. The polysaccharide is absorbed by the cell, as may be demonstrated by specific antiserum. Red blood cells which have absorbed inhibitor will still adsorb virus but will not agglutinate. In other words, these inhibitors influence virus multiplication independent of any effect on hemagglutination. One might say that in the Hirst phenomenon the competition between inhibitor and virus is for union with the cell. In the second case, the competition is *within* the cell.

Although the influence of different polysaccharides on the relationship between various viruses and cells is at present unpredictable, the occurrence of such substances may be of great moment in prophylaxis and therapy. What part inhibitors play in modifying the occurrence and course of natural infections and in contributing to the great diversity of clinical symptoms we do not know. But since inhibitors are found in "normal" animals, their occurrence may be commonplace, whatever their effect. One example of what may occur is provided by the plant pathologists. Our knowledge of virus diseases of plants has closely paralleled that of virus diseases of animals, and it is not surprising that plant pathologists also have discovered the existence of inhibitory substances. Thus Doolittle and Walker (17) discovered that they could not recover cucumber mosaic virus from poleweed leaves because of an inhibitor in the plant juices but that infection was easily transmitted by aphids. One might remember this when confronted with a troublesome isolation or evidence of transmission by unusual means. Recently an inhibitor in normal allantoic fluid was described (18, 19). This substance, probably a mucoprotein, is capable of combining with influenza virus and when released is no longer capable of further combination. Virus combined with the inhibitor is infectious and combines with red blood cells without causing agglutination. Contamination of highly purified influenza preparations with this substance must be considered. Some years ago Traub (20) observed that choriomeningitis virus vaccines prepared from heterologous tissues were unsatisfactory. Organ extracts from other species also inhibited their action. Similar observations have been made in the case of distemper (21) and influenza vaccines (22). We may anticipate that our present knowledge of virus inhibitors is but a beginning and that a much better understanding of the relations between viruses and cells will come from a continuation of this already profitable research.

Having avoided structural blockades, antisera, and inhibitors, the virus must yet find a suitable cell. To be suitable, the cell must frequently be of a particular tissue of an appropriate animal species. In addition, the age of the animal may be important. The differences which exist between the cells of different species and tissues are crucial to the virus, but we know little about them. On the whole, it seems that the differences are often relative and may be overcome by the experimenter if he provides sufficient opportunities for the virus to adapt itself to the new conditions. Even our conception of the host range and neurotropism of poliomyelitis virus, which have appeared to be conspicuously rigid, are slowly being modified.

Indeed, it seems that the possibilities of adapting viruses to other species are considerable and better techniques may yield many surprises. Baker (23), for example, adapted rinderpest and hog cholera to the rabbit by alternate passages in susceptible and resistant animals. We have adapted the OT strain of mouse encephalomyelitis virus to hamsters by this method (24). Here, as in many other instances, there was evidence of a rather sudden change in the virus itself, a change usually characterized as a mutation. In our experiments the change occurred after several generations and then remained fixed; that is, hamster pathogenicity has persisted ever since. Interestingly, the modified virus will cause paralysis in hamsters only if it has recently been passaged in mice. A single mouse passage will completely restore pathogenicity to the modified virus, whereas several passages were required initially. It may be that alternate passages, by maintaining the concentration of the virus, simply provide a means of multiplying the opportunities necessary to the occurrence of a successful mutant. If this is so, equal success might follow if one inoculated a large number of the resistant species at one time. However valid these explanations may prove to be, the frequent occurrence of adaptation is well established and may at times be of great importance in nature. You will remember that Theobald Smith (25) believed that mutations are often the cause of epidemics. Recently a start has been made in studying bacterial viruses by the methods geneticists use. The initial observations support the theory that mutations do occur (26). However, we should remember that a corollary may exist between viruses and adaptive enzymes. Yeast and bacteria have both yielded fractions which stimulate the growth of phage (27).

If something of this kind also occurs with animal viruses, we should look to the host cell as well as to the virus for the factors responsible for adaptations.

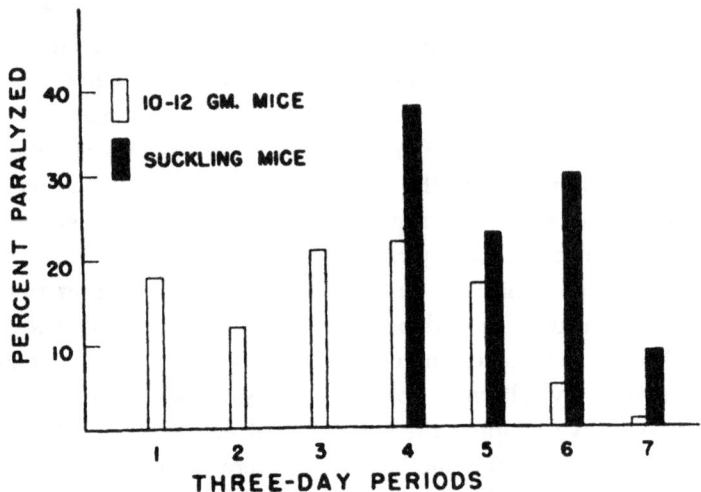

THE INCUBATION PERIOD OF LANSING POLIOMYELITIS IN SUCKLING MICE

Age plays a significant role in certain virus diseases. Olitsky and his associates (28) explored this subject after observing that only immature mice are susceptible to intraperitoneally injected vesicular stomatitis virus. Their work established that barriers to the spread of certain viruses develop with increasing age. In older mice, virus introduced into the eye was stopped by the retina, virus injected into the muscles of an extremity remained there, and that instilled into the nostrils did not extend beyond the olfactory area of the brain.

We have recently found evidence of an age factor which may be a property of the cell itself. This came about while studying the agent recovered last year from the feces of paralyzed children (29). The virus is unique in that it paralyzes only suckling mice and hamsters, irrespective of the route of inoculation. Animals ten to twelve days old are usually resistant. We have injected several other viruses in suckling mice. When the mouse-adapted Lansing strain of poliomyelitis virus is used, the reverse occurs and the mice do not become paralyzed until they have matured. The incubation period is lengthened by ten or more days. (See figure.) It would seem that susceptibility to the first agent disappears at the time it develops to the second. I do not consider such an observation to be particularly surprising. Cells are born, age, and die, and their metabolic processes presumably undergo many changes, just as their appearance does. But we must remember that some viruses are dependent on the maturation of their hosts.

Each of these variables having been resolved in favor of union of virus and cell, there may still remain other qualifying conditions. The cell may be exposed and of the proper kind, and still not be receptive. It may be unreceptive because it is already occupied by another virus. This is the basis of the "interference phenomenon," which was first recognized as "a new immunity mechanism" in 1937 (30), although the protective or curative effect of one disease on another had long been known to clinicians. Edward Jenner (31) described "modification of vaccinia pustule occasioned by an herpetic state of the skin" in 1804, and Thomas Archer (32), the mitigating effect of vaccinia on "the hooping cough" in 1809. Moreover, drug interferences were clearly recognized by Browning and Gulbransen (33) in 1922, and Magrassi (34) in 1935 described conditions under which the intracutaneous inoculation of herpes virus afforded transient immunity to an intracerebral challenge.

From the beginning, it was appreciated that only certain viruses conflict. (See Tables 1 and 2.) Thus, monkeys survived the inoculation of poliomyelitis virus if they had previously been injected with a suspension of dog distemper spleen, but they died like controls when vaccinia and eastern equine encephalomyelitis viruses were used (35). Later it was learned that distemper preparation itself was a mixture of distemper and choriomeningitis viruses, of which only the latter interferes with poliomyelitis (36). Nor did the distemper and choriomeningitis viruses interfere with one another. The mixture had been maintained through many generations over many years without loss of either. At about the same time Syverton and Berry (37) demonstrated that cells containing papilloma virus could be superinfected with other viruses and that the inclusion bodies of two different diseases might be found to occur simultaneously in single cells. Thus it seemed all the more likely that interference is a rather selective form of biologic competition and is limited to special combinations. It should be noted that this may not be true of bacterial viruses.

Delbrück (38) writes that "exclusion occurs between any pair of viruses which has been tested, whether the viruses are related or not." It would seem that this observation is inapplicable to animal

TABLE 1

INTERFERENCE BETWEEN ANIMAL VIRUSES

HETEROLOGOUS

Rift Valley fever	Yellow fever	Findlay and MacCallum (1937)
Choriomeningitis	Poliomyelitis	Dalldorf et al. (1937)
Virus III	Shope fibroma	Andrewes (1940)
W. E. encephalomyelitis	E. E. encephalomyelitis	Schlesinger et al. (1943–44)
W. E. encephalomyelitis	Vesicular stomatitis	Schlesinger et al. (1943–44)
Mouse encephalomyelitis	W. E. encephalomyelitis	Schlesinger et al. (1943–44)
Influenza viruses		Henle and Henle (1943)
		Ziegler et al. (1944)
St. Louis encephalitis	W. E. encephalomyelitis	Duffy (1944)
W. E. encephalomyelitis	Influenza	Henle and Henle (1945)
Keratoconjunctivitis	Influenza	Henle and Henle (1945)
Mumps	W. E. encephalomyelitis	Henle and Henle (1945)
Yellow fever	West Nile	Lennette and Koprowski (1946)
Yellow fever	E. enceph. (Venez.)	Lennette and Koprowski (1946)
Papilloma	Sheep dermatitis	Selbie (1946)
Vaccinia	Ectromelia	Andrewes and Elford (1947)
Influenza	Yellow fever	Vilches and Hirst (1947)
Influenza	Rabies	Vilches and Hirst (1947)
Influenza	Semliki Forest	Vilches and Hirst (1947)
Influenza	Newcastle	Ginsberg and Horsfall (1948)

TABLE 2

INTERFERENCE BETWEEN ANIMAL VIRUSES

HOMOLOGOUS

Sheep pox	Donatien (1932)
Yellow fever	Hoskins (1935)
Herpes	Magrassi (1935)
Phage	White (1937)
Influenza	Rickard and Francis (1938)
Rinderpest	Pfaff (1938)
Poliomyelitis	Jungeblut and Sanders (1940)
Distemper	Green and Stulberg (1946)
Ectromelia	Andrewes and Elford (1947)
Vaccinia	Dalldorf, Cohen, and Coffey (1947)

viruses, although the failure to interfere in animal experiments may simply be due to the fact that the two agents do not engage identical cells, as they must in the case of the simpler phage experiments.

The critical importance of time was also evident from the first interference experiments. The two infections had to be combined after certain intervals. Furthermore, the phenomenon could readily be dissociated from the effects of biologically inert particulate matter which Ledingham (39) had found influenced the development of the vaccinia lesion by reticulo-endothelial blockade. And it was shown to be little, if at all, dependent on inflammation. Since the initial experiments, instances have been found in which the interference is wholly local, and evidence has accumulated that the first agent does not simply accelerate the formation of immune substance, for interference has been induced within one minute and is relatively nonspecific. Indeed, humoral immunity seems to play no part whatever in the interference phenomenon. Whether species ever plays a role, I do not know. In general, it has been true that every animal species susceptible to both viruses will show a degree of interference, although we could not transpose to mice what worked so well in monkeys, and Vilches and Hirst (40) mention a failure to duplicate in fertile eggs what succeeded in mice.

These are the chief characteristics of interference between viruses. The phenomenon has had little application outside of research, yet clues to its presence may be detected elsewhere. Doubtless it has in the past sometimes led to experimental errors. Browning and Gulbransen's suggestion (41) that in the case of drugs great care is necessary in drawing conclusions as to the therapeutic efficacy of impure preparations because of the possibility that isomers may be present and interfere, doubtless has application in virology as well. An unsuspected interference may occur when a contaminating second virus is present or when some of the virus is attenuated but nevertheless able to interfere. The conflict between active and inactive virus of the same kind has been called "auto-interference." Thus the Henles (42) found that inactive virus accumulated in allantoic fluids infected with influenza virus, and, when these were transferred as concentrated inocula to chick embryos, the yield of virus was low because of an interference. Interference must be considered in cross-immunity tests, and Andrewes and Elford (43) suggest that certain vaccines are interfering rather than immunizing agents.

I have looked for evidence that interference has epidemiologic importance. The report by Findlay and MacCallum (44) of interference between Rift Valley fever and yellow fever mentions the distribution of the two diseases in Africa, which is quite different. The authors were seeking relationships between the two viruses. Possibly the difference in distribution reflects an interference in nature. Recently Stephens (45) has described an epidemic of atypical pneumonia in an area in which infectious hepatitis was endemic, and noted that no new cases of hepatitis were seen during the epidemic, although they recurred once it ceased.

Interference has been applied in the treatment of canine distemper. An attenuated distemper virus is used to modify the natural infection (46). It has been suggested that the interference phenomenon may be used in diagnosing the presence of poliomyelitis virus by first inoculating mice with a suspension of patient's feces and shortly afterward challenging with a mouse-adapted strain of virus (47, 48).

A number of explanations of the interference phenomenon have been proposed. I have arranged the principal ones in Table 3. It is

Table 3
Interference Phenomenon Hypotheses

I. "Cellular blockade" (44) Cell receptor blockade (49)	Not simply blockade, since some inactivated viruses are adsorbed but no longer interfere.
II. Competition for cell nutrient, (35) destruction of particular substrate, or enzyme blockade within cell (40)	Not demonstrated. Related to resistance of sick animals and those on deficient diets.
III. Formation of a poorly diffusible inhibitory substance within cell (50)	Inhibitor not demonstrated.
IV. "Penetration hypothesis," (51) analogous to sperm-ova union	Suggested by electron microscope studies. Necessary to postulate excluded virus may still compete for cell substrate.
V. Genetic (52)	Competition similar to II, exaggerated by tendency of two to hybridize, resulting in many nonviable forms of secondary agent.

likely, as others have suggested (40), that more than one mechanism is involved. It is also quite evident that those mechanisms which have been disclosed through studies of virus hemagglutination may be equally applicable to virus interference, and the two lines of investigation are now converging.

There are additional mechanisms by which cells become nonreceptive to viruses. Surely something should be said of cellular immunity. Francis (53) clearly separated humoral and tissue immunity in experimental influenza. In many diseases the influence of antibodies is difficult to assess, although there is evidence of an independent immunity.

It might be well to try to relate cell immunity to some of the things we have already considered—the presence of inhibitors, the persistence of virus. The persistence of virus has long been considered a possible explanation of persistent immunity but proof is difficult. Obviously, if virus persisted—and Shope has shown how inadequate our tests for its presence may be—persistence immunity could be due to an interference as well as to the constant stimulation of humoral antibodies. On this point we have no conclusive evidence as yet, but I think it interesting to note that the union of virus with cells may be dependent on other immune mechanisms than those we have known so long. For there are a variety of observations which point to additional phenomena. I would like to mention three which have much interested us.

It is known that rabbit papilloma virus tends to disappear from the tumors of domesticated rabbits. Bernheim (54) found in such tumors an enzyme which hydrolyzes papilloma virus. If this be considered an acquired cellular immunity, it obviously is a very special kind.

Gard (55) showed that suspensions of the brain tissue of mice which had survived an attack of encephalomyelitis prevent infection when injected with active virus. No evidence of interference was found and the agent did not combine with the virus *in vitro*. The protective substance was not a globulin. It was associated with the tissue itself and was insoluble in water and saline. This, too, suggests an acquired immunity of a special kind.

We have investigated an inhibitor which occurs in the feces of very old mice and which inactivates mouse encephalomyelitis virus (56). As you know, most mouse colonies are infected with this virus, which

Theiler discovered (57) and Olitsky (58) showed is excreted in the feces. We find that as mice become old they cease to excrete virus. Their feces then contain an inhibitor which may be demonstrated by mixing fecal suspensions with virus and titrating the mixture in mice. For a time we suspected that antibody was excreted by the bowel wall, as occurs in cholera and dysentery (59, 60). That explanation now seems unlikely. For one thing, the inhibitor effect is greatly increased with prolonged incubation, and globulins have not been separable from the suspensions. Furthermore, our tests do not show a close correlation between serum antibody and fecal inhibitor, and hyperimmunization of mice, which leads to high titers of humoral antibody, does not stop the fecal excretion of virus in younger animals. The lipid fraction has so far been inactive. Apparently the agent is associated with coarse particulate material, and the best concentrations so far achieved have been through fractional centrifugation. The fecal inhibitor is in this respect similar to the tissue component Gard described, but the method of its *in vitro* action is different and more nearly resembles the effect of an enzyme.

These are but random samples from a long and growing list of observations which suggest additional mechanisms that influence the relationships between viruses and cells. It would be foolhardy to predict where the trail will eventually lead, but it should bring us closer to the heart of the problem where knowledge of great fundamental value lies.

REFERENCES

1. Kidd, J. G., The enduring partnership of a neoplastic virus and carcinoma cells, *J. Exp. Med.*, 1942, 75:7.
2. Rous, Peyton, P. D. McMaster, and S. S. Hudack, The fixation and protection of viruses by the cells of susceptible animals, *J. Exp. Med.*, 1935, 61:657.
3. Andrewes, C. H., Anti-vaccinial serum, 1: Protection against generalisations in the rabbit, 2: The time factor in protection experiments, *J. Path. & Bact.*, 1929, 32:265.
4. Olitsky, P. K., and A. B. Sabin, Comparative effectiveness of various chemical sprays in protecting monkeys against nasally instilled poliomyelitis virus, *Proc. Soc. Exp. Biol. & Med.*, 1937, 36:532.
5. Armstrong, Charles, Studies on the mechanism of experimental intranasal infection in mice, *Pub. Health Rep.*, 1938, 53:2004.

6. Hirst, G. K., Adsorption of influenza hemagglutinins and virus by red blood cells, *J. Exp. Med.*, 1942, 76:195.
7. Lanni, Frank, and J. W. Beard, The mechanism of egg-white inhibition of hemagglutination by swine influenza virus, *Proc. Soc. Exp. Biol. & Med.*, 1948, 68:442.
8. Hirst, G. K., The nature of the virus receptors of red cells, I: Evidence on the chemical nature of the virus receptors of red cells and of the existence of a closely analogous substance in normal serum, *J. Exp. Med.*, 1948, 87:301.
9. Burnet, F. M., and J. D. Stone, The receptor-destroying enzyme of V. cholerae, *Australian J. Exp. Biol. & Med. Sci.*, 1947, 25:227. Burnet, F. M., The initiation of cellular infection by influenza and related viruses, *Lancet*, 1948, 254:7.
10. Anderson, S. G., The mechanism of the union between influenza virus and susceptible cells, *Australian J. Sci.*, 1947, 10:83.
11. Burnet, F. M., J. F. McCrea, and J. D. Stone, Modification of human red cells by virus action, I: The receptor gradient for virus action in human red cells, *Brit. J. Exp. Path.*, 1946, 27:228.
12. Bovarnick, Max, and P. M. de Burgh, Virus hemagglutination, *Science*, 1947, 105:550.
13. de Burgh, P. M., P-C. Yu, Calderon Howe, and Max Bovarnick, Preparation from human red cells of a substance inhibiting virus hemagglutination, *J. Exp. Med.*, 1948, 87:1.
14. Friedewald, W. F., E. S. Miller, and L. R. Whatley, The nature of nonspecific inhibition of virus hemagglutination, *J. Exp. Med.*, 1947, 86:65.
15. Ginsberg, H. S., W. F. Goebel, and F. L. Horsfall, Jr., The inhibitory effect of polysaccharide on mumps virus multiplication, *J. Exp. Med.*, 1948, 87:385.
16. Horsfall, F. L., Jr., and Maclyn McCarty, The modifying effects of certain substances of bacterial origin on the course of infection with pneumonia virus of mice (PVM), *J. Exp. Med.*, 1947, 85:623.
17. Doolittle, S. P., and M. N. Walker, Further studies on the overwintering and dissemination of curcurbit mosaic, *J. Agr. Res.* 1925, 31:1.
18. Magill, T. P., and J. Y. Sugg, Physical-chemical factors in agglutination of sheep erythrocytes by influenza virus, *Proc. Soc. Exp. Biol. & Med.*, 1947, 66:89.
19. Hardy, P. H., Jr., and F. L. Horsfall, Jr., Reactions between influenza virus and a component of allantoic fluid, *J. Exp. Med.*, 1948, 88:463.
20. Traub, Erich, Immunization of guinea pigs against lymphocytic choriomeningitis with formolized tissue vaccines, *J. Exp. Med.*, 1938, 68:95.
21. Laidlaw, P. P., and G. W. Dunkin, Studies in dog distemper; immunization of dogs, *J. Comp. Path. & Therap.*, 1928, 41:209.
22. Andrewes, C. H., and Wilson Smith, The effect of foreign tissue extracts on the efficacy of influenza virus vaccines, *Brit. J. Exp. Path.*, 1939, 20:305.

23. Baker, J. A., Serial passage of hog cholera virus in rabbits, *Proc. Soc. Exp. Biol. & Med.*, 1946, 63:183.
 ——— Rinderpest infection in rabbits, *Am. J. Vet. Res.*, 1946, 7:179.
24. Dean, D. J., and Gilbert Dalldorf, The susceptibility of the hamster to mouse encephalomyelitis, *J. Exp. Med.*, 1948, 88:645.
25. Smith, Theobald, *Parasitism and Disease* (Princeton University Press, 1934). 196 pp.
26. Hershey, A. D., and Raquel Rotman, Linkage among genes controlling inhibition of lysis in a bacterial virus, *Proc. Nat. Acad. Sci.*, 1948, 34:89.
27. Price, W. H., The stimulatory action of certain fractions from bacteria and yeast on the formation of a bacterial virus, *Proc. Nat. Acad. Sci.*, 1948, 34:317.
28. Olitsky, P. K., and J. Casals, Concepts of the immunology of certain virus infections, *Bull. New York Acad. Med.*, 1945, 21:356.
29. Dalldorf, Gilbert, and G. M. Sickles, An unidentified, filterable agent isolated from the feces of children with paralysis, *Science*, 1948, 108:61.
30. Dalldorf, Gilbert, Margaret Douglass, and H. E. Robinson, The sparing effect of dog distemper on experimental poliomyelitis, *Science*, 1937, 85:184.
31. Jenner, Edward, On the varieties and modifications of the vaccine pustule, occasioned by an herpetic state of the skin, *Med. & Phys. J.*, August, 1804, 41, No. 66.
32. Archer, John, The hooping-cough cured by vaccination, *Med. Repository*, 1809, 6:182.
33. Browning, C. H., and R. Gulbransen, An interference phenomenon in the action of chemotherapeutic substances in experimental trypanosome infections, *J. Path. & Bact.*, 1922, 25:395.
34. Magrassi, Flaviano, Studii sull'infezione e sull'immunit' da virus erpetico, *Zeit. f. Hyg. und Infekt.*, 1935, 117:573.
35. Dalldorf, Gilbert, Margaret Douglass, and H. E. Robinson, The sparing effect of canine distemper on poliomyelitis in macaca mulatta, *J. Exp. Med.*, 1938, 67:333.
36. Dalldorf, Gilbert, The simultaneous occurrence of the viruses of canine distemper and lymphocytic choriomeningitis, *J. Exp. Med.*, 1939, 70:19.
37. Syverton, J. T., and G. P. Berry, The superinfection of the rabbit papilloma (Shope) by extraneous viruses, *J. Exp. Med.*, 1947, 86:131.
 ——— Multiple virus infection of single host cells, *J. Exp. Med.*, 1947, 86:145.
38. Delbrück, M., Biochemical mutants of bacterial viruses, *J. Bact.*, 1948, 56:1.
39. Ledingham, J. C. G., The role of the reticulo-endothelial system of the cutis in experimental vaccinia and other infections: Experiments with India ink, *Brit. J. Exp. Path.*, 1927, 8:12.
40. Vilches, Antonio, and G. K. Hirst, Interference between neurotropic and other unrelated viruses, *J. Immunol.*, 1947, 57:125.

41. Browning, C. H., and others, Therapeutic interference caused by isomerides of trypanocidal styryl quinoline derivatives, *Proc. Roy. Soc., s.B.*, London, 1931, 109:51.
42. Henle, Werner, and Gertrude Henle, Interference of inactive virus with the propagation of virus of influenza, *Science*, 1943, 98:87.
    ——— Interference between inactive and active viruses of influenza, I: The incidental occurrence and artificial induction of the phenomenon, II: Factors influencing the phenomenon, *Am. J. Med. Sci.*, 1944, 207:705, 717.
43. Andrewes, C. H., and W. J. Elford, Infectious ectromelia: Experiments on interference and immunization, *Brit. J. Exp. Path.*, 1947, 28:278.
44. Findlay, G. M., and F. O. MacCallum, An interference phenomenon in relation to yellow fever and other viruses, *J. Path. & Bact.*, 1937, 44:405.
45. Stephens, J. W., Primary atypical pneumonia, *Lancet*, 1948, 254:703.
46. Green, R. G., and C. S. Stulberg, Cell-blockade in canine distemper, *Proc. Soc. Exp. Biol. & Med.*, 1946, 61:117.
47. Dalldorf, Gilbert, and Elinor Whitney, A further interference in experimental poliomyelitis, *Science*, 1943, 98:477.
48. Lépine, P. R., A laboratory test for the virus of poliomyelitis, *Science*, 1948, 108:134.
49. White, P. B., Lysogenic strains of V. cholerae and the influence of lysozyme on cholera phage activity, *J. Path. & Bact.*, 1937, 44:276.
50. Andrewes, C. H., Interference by one virus with the growth of another in tissue-culture, *Brit. J. Exp. Path.*, 1942, 23:214.
51. Delbrück, M., Interference between bacterial viruses, III: The mutual exclusion effect and the depressor effect, *J. Bact.*, 1945, 50:151.
52. Hershey, A. D., and J. Bronfenbrenner, Bacterial viruses, bacteriophages, in *Viral and Rickettsial Infections of Man*, T. M. Rivers, ed., pp. 147–162 (Philadelphia, J. B. Lippincott Co., 1948).
53. Francis, Thomas, Jr., The significance of nasal factors in epidemic influenza. In Bicentennial Conference of Pennsylvania University: Problems and Trends in Virus Research, Philadelphia, 1941, pp. 41–54.
54. Bernheim, Frederick, M. L. C. Bernheim, A. R. Taylor, Dorothy Beard, D. G. Sharp, and J. W. Beard, A factor in domestic rabbit papilloma tissue hydrolyzing the papilloma virus protein, *Science*, 1942, 95:230.
55. Gard, S., Tissue immunity in mouse poliomyelitis, *Acta Med. Scandinav.* 1944, 119:27.
56. Dalldorf, Gilbert, and D. J. Dean, An encephalomyelitis virus inhibitor in mouse feces, *Proc. IV. Internat. Congress for Microbiology* (1947). Copenhagen, 1949, p. 252.
57. Theiler, Max, Spontaneous encephalomyelitis of mice, a new virus disease, *J. Exp. Med.*, 1937, 65:705.
58. Olitsky, P. K., A transmissible agent (Theiler's virus) in the intestines of normal mice, *J. Exp. Med.*, 1940, 72:113.

59. Davies, Arthur, An investigation into the serological properties of dysentery stools, *Lancet*, 1922, 203:1009.
60. Burrows, William, M. E. Elliott, and Isabelle Havens, Studies on immunity to Asiatic cholera, IV: The excretion of coproantibody in experimental enteric cholera in the guinea pig, *J. Infect. Dis.*, 1947, 81:261.

Chapter 5

THE ACTIVATION OF VIRUSES BY ADSORPTION COFACTORS[1]

By THOMAS F. ANDERSON, *Johnson Foundation, University of Pennsylvania*

I SHALL DESCRIBE experiments on the pathogenesis and pathology of virus diseases not of man nor even of animals but of bacteria, and attempt to point out the significance of the results to the general science of virology. As you are all well aware, the etiological agents of virus diseases of bacteria are called bacteriophages or bacterial viruses. These viruses may produce lysis of all the susceptible cells in a broth culture, or, if the growing bacteria are immobilized on a solid medium such as agar, each particle may initiate the formation of a localized lytic area or plaque on the bacterial smear, quite analogous to the "pocks" which certain animal viruses form on the skin or on the membranes of the chick embryo. Counts of the number of plaques which suitable dilutions of bacteriophage form on a bacterial smear provide estimates of the concentration of active particles accurate to within 10 percent.

A single strain of a bacterium such as *Escherichia coli* may be susceptible to a hundred or more demonstrably different strains of virus. A group of workers in this country has chosen to concentrate its attention on a set of seven viruses collected by Demerec and Fano (1) at Cold Spring Harbor and all active on a single strain B of *E. coli*. These seven strains were serially designated $T_1, T_2, \ldots T_7$, "T" standing for "type."

When examined in the electron microscope (2) it turned out that the even-numbered viruses, T_2, T_4, and T_6, have identical morphologies, being tadpole-shaped, with the head, about 0.08μ in diameter, consisting of internal structures surrounded by a membrane to which

---

[1] This work was supported by Contract N6 ori 168 TO II between the Office of Naval Research and the Trustees of the University of Pennsylvania and the Government is hereby granted royalty-free right of reproduction.

a well-defined tail is attached. Parenthetically, I might mention that vaccinia virus, too, has a membrane surrounding internal structures, but as far as we know, it has no tail. T_3 and T_7 also seem identical, being little spheres only 0.04μ in diameter. The remaining two are dissimilar. T_1 has a small head 0.045μ in diameter to which a faint tail is attached, while T_5 has a large, almost empty head about 0.1μ in diameter with a long tail attached to it. Morphologicaly, these viruses thus fall into four distinct groups.

Serologicaly the classification is the same. Antisera against T_1 or against T_5 react with none of the other viruses, while antisera against T_3 inactivate T_7. Antisera against T_2 inactivate T_4 and T_6. It thus seems probable that T_2 is related phylogenetically to T_4 and T_6 and that T_3 is related to T_7 (3).

The bacteriophages which have been analyzed chemically seem to resemble the animal viruses more than they do the plant viruses, for their nucleic acids are of the desoxypentose type, like that of the animal viruses. The plant viruses, in contrast, all contain nucleic acids of the pentose rather than the desoxypentose variety (2).

So much for the virus particles. They are inert, stable bodies which survive years of storage in the refrigerator. It is only when they come in contact with their particular host cell that they show physiological activity. Then their behavior seems to be similar in many respects to that of the viruses of animals. They exhibit, first of all, the interference phenomenon between two unrelated viruses infecting the same host cell. Their life cycle consists of three easily recognizable stages (4): first, adsorption on the host cell; second, vegetative growth within the host cell; and third, liberation from the host cell in a burst of a hundred or more daughter particles, which may then infect other host cells in the neighborhood. This life cycle is duplicated by influenza virus growing on the chick embryo, as recently reported by Dr. and Mrs. Henle and Miss Rosenberg (5) at the Children's Hospital in Philadelphia.

More recent research on the life cycles of bacterial viruses has revealed many new and unexpected details in the above picture. I shall tell you about some of them. Perhaps they will assist in understanding the behavior of those viruses which infect certain groups of cells in those complex colonies of differentiated cells which we call animals and plants.

The effects of adsorption of virus on *E. coli* are cataclysmic, for once a virus like T_2 is adsorbed on the cell, the processes of growth of the cell stop abruptly (6). This is most strikingly brought out by recent work at the Pasteur Institute by Monod and Wollman (7), who find that once a virus is adsorbed, the host cell cannot adapt its metabolism to use a sugar which was absent from the medium in which growth of the cell had taken place. Since normal cells can readily synthesize the new enzymes required for such a conversion of metabolism, it would appear that the virus blocks the synthesis of such enzymes. These viruses seem to cancel the synthetic processes of the host cell and convert them to the synthesis of more virus.

We are obtaining a few clues to the mechanism of virus production within the host cell. Dr. A. H. Doermann and I (report unpublished) have broken open cells with sonic vibration at various times after infection with T_3 and have determined the number of particles present before lysis would normally have occurred. For some time after infection no virus could be recovered, not even the one which had infected the cell. This particle must have changed its state in some way, for free T_3 particles are quite resistant to sonic vibration. Suddenly, however, at 12 minutes after infection, and well before lysis would normally have occurred, virus began to be produced rapidly, until the cells began to liberate virus by the normal process of lysis at 18 minutes. These results confirm those which Doermann had obtained previously, using different methods in studying the multiplication of T_4, and suggest that the greatly dissimilar viruses T_3 and T_4 multiply by similar processes. These processes seem to involve a labile, vegetative state which sets the stage for the synthesis of mature virus particles.

Some of the most striking results have been obtained by those studying the genetic properties of bacterial viruses. Mutations in bacterial viruses are now well known and affect such properties as host range, plaque morphology, and, as I shall have occasion to mention later, cofactor requirements. And so there is available for study a whole series of forms containing mutant genes in many combinations suitable for the study of genetic crosses between virus strains.

It was in 1945 that Hershey (8) observed the breakdown of the then all-embracing interference phenomenon. He infected cells of *E. coli* simultaneously with two strains of T_2, one of which formed fuzzy plaques and the other, clear plaques. Individual cells with this mixed infection produced both types of virus; therefore, both must have multiplied within the same host cell or one virus caused some of the other to adopt its character.

A better understanding of this breakdown of the interference phenomenon arises from experiments in which bacteria are infected simultaneously with two related viruses which differ from each other in many respects. In this case, too, both the infecting types are recovered in the offspring, but virus particles containing the genetic traits of the parent particles in various new combinations are also present. The parent viruses have crossed to produce hybrid types! As Hershey has pointed out, "This sort of hybridization may serve in nature to multiply the seemingly unlimited array of existing types of virus." Such crosses have been observed between the related viruses T_2, T_4, and T_6, but not with the others. By analyses of the frequency of such exchanges Hershey and Rotman (9) have been able to establish linkage groups for the different characters and assign the genes involved to positions on gene maps analogous to those made by Morgan and his school for the genes of the fruit fly *Drosophila*.

These, then, are some of the consequences of the adsorption of these viruses on their host cells. The cofactor phenomenon which I shall now describe provides the first faint clue to the mechanism by which a virus is brought from a state of indifference to its surroundings to one in which it is not only able but apparently eager to initiate such phenomena as these.

Some years ago, in studying the multiplication of the virus T_2 on ultraviolet-irradiated host cells I employed a growth medium containing ammonium lactate as the source of nitrogen and carbon. This medium had the advantage of being transparent to the ultraviolet. The bacteria grew well on this medium, and T_2 formed plaques on bacterial smears growing on agar containing this limited nutrient with the same efficiency as it did on agar containing the richest nutrients. In this medium T_2 even grew well on bacteria which had been killed many times over with ultraviolet light (10).

In attempting to extend these studies to T_2's distant cousins, T_4 (Fig. 1) and T_6, we found (11) that certain stocks of these viruses were most inefficient in forming plaques on the bacteria grown on ammonium lactate, as compared to nutrient agar, which contained an

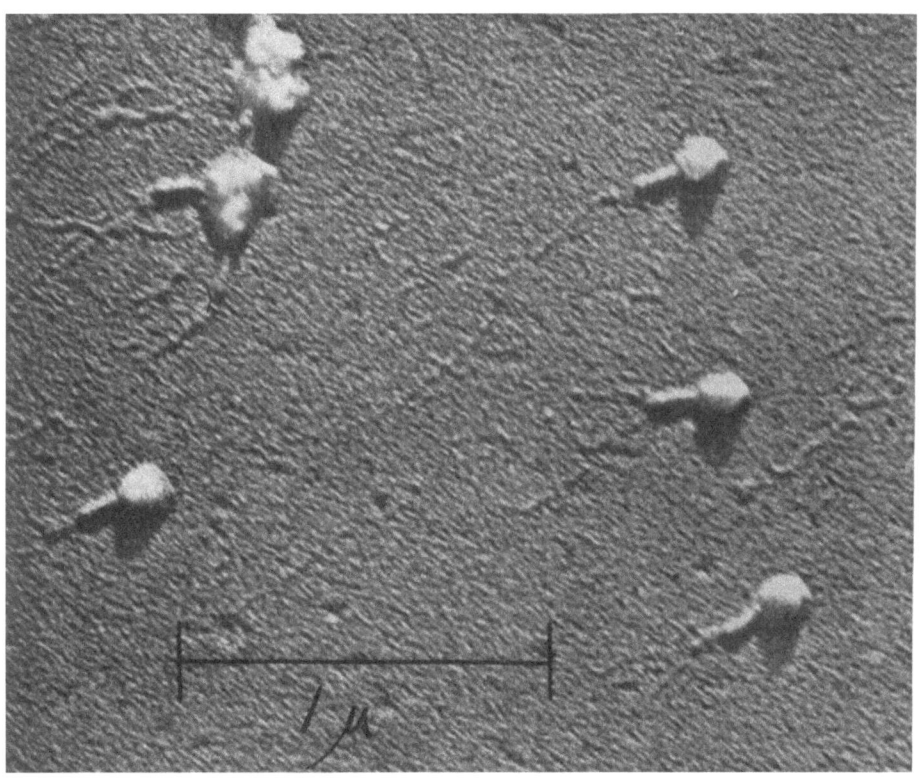

FIGURE 1. THE BACTERIAL VIRUS T$_4$, PURIFIED AND SHADOWED WITH GOLD AS SEEN IN THE ELECTRON MICROSCOPE
Magnification = × 50,000. EMG 199b.

abundance of growth factors and amino acids. We therefore turned to a study of the peculiar behavior of these stocks in which a nutritional deficiency involving the virus activity seemed to exist in the ammonium-lactate medium. By testing each of the amino acids and growth factors individually it was found that the addition of minute amounts of L-tryptophan, larger amounts of phenylalanine or diiodotyrosine, or still larger amounts of tyrosine to the ammonium-lactate agar promoted plaque formation by both the viruses, T_4 and T_6. None of the other natural amino acids or growth factors tested had this effect. It was readily shown by use of the electron microscope (Figs. 2, 3) and the centrifuge that without one of these substances as cofactor these viruses were not even adsorbed on the host cell. The cofactor phenomenon therefore concerns the initiation of the virus attack on the host cell. We may express these phenomena in other terms: the host cells are resistant to these stocks of T_4 and T_6 in ammonium-lactate medium, but they are sensitive if cofactor is added to the medium.

The essential feature of the cofactor molecule is the L-amino-acid grouping, for any change in this group in L-tryptophan, such as substitution or conversion to the D form, destroyed its activity. On the other hand, rather radical changes in the aromatic group yielded compounds with decreased, but still measurable, activities (2) (Table 1). One of these compounds, 5-methyltryptophan, is of particular interest in this connection, for in the minimal medium it proved (12) to have a bacteriostatic action which could be reversed by traces of tryptophan. Still, 5-methyltryptophan is a perfectly good cofactor in promoting the adsorption of T_4 on its host cell.

Two other cofactors are of special interest—2-pyridylalanine and 3-pyridylalanine. They promoted adsorption of the viruses on the host cells, but if allowed to remain in the medium during multiplication of the virus they inhibited the formation of plaques by the virus (2). They thus fulfilled the requirements of an antiviral agent: they inhibited virus growth while allowing host cells to multiply.

The question now arises: Do the cofactors act on the host cells in making them more "receptive" to the virus or on the virus in making it more readily adsorbed on the host? Many experiments have shown that the cofactor exerts its action on the virus particle (13). For example, if T_4 is equilibrated with 2 micrograms of L-tryptophan per

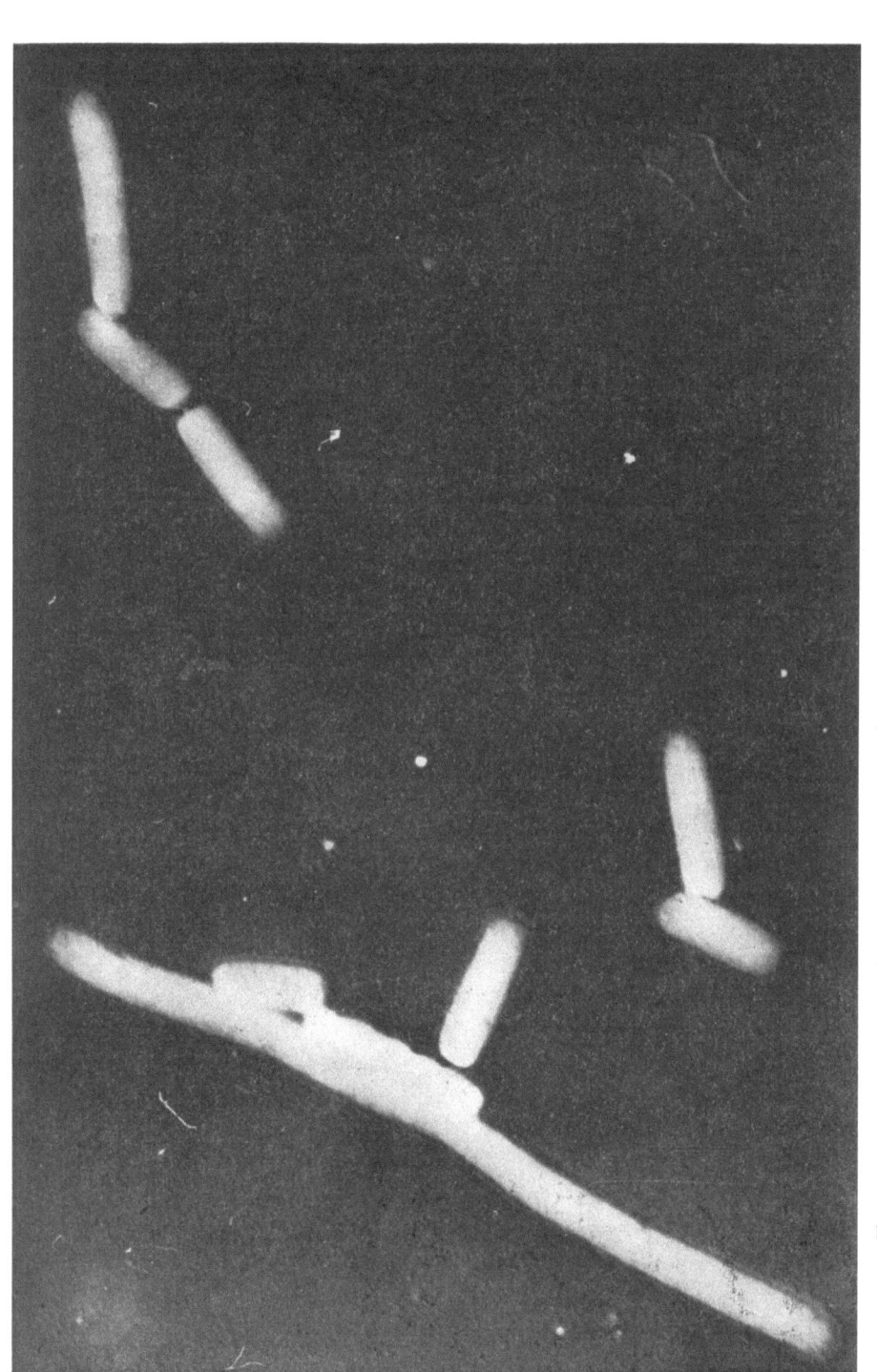

FIGURE 2. AN ELECTRON MICROGRAPH OF *E. coli* STRAIN B WHICH HAD BEEN EXPOSED TO THE VIRUS T4 IN THE ABSENCE OF ADDED COFACTOR

It can be seen that no virus has been adsorbed on the cells. EMG 213d.

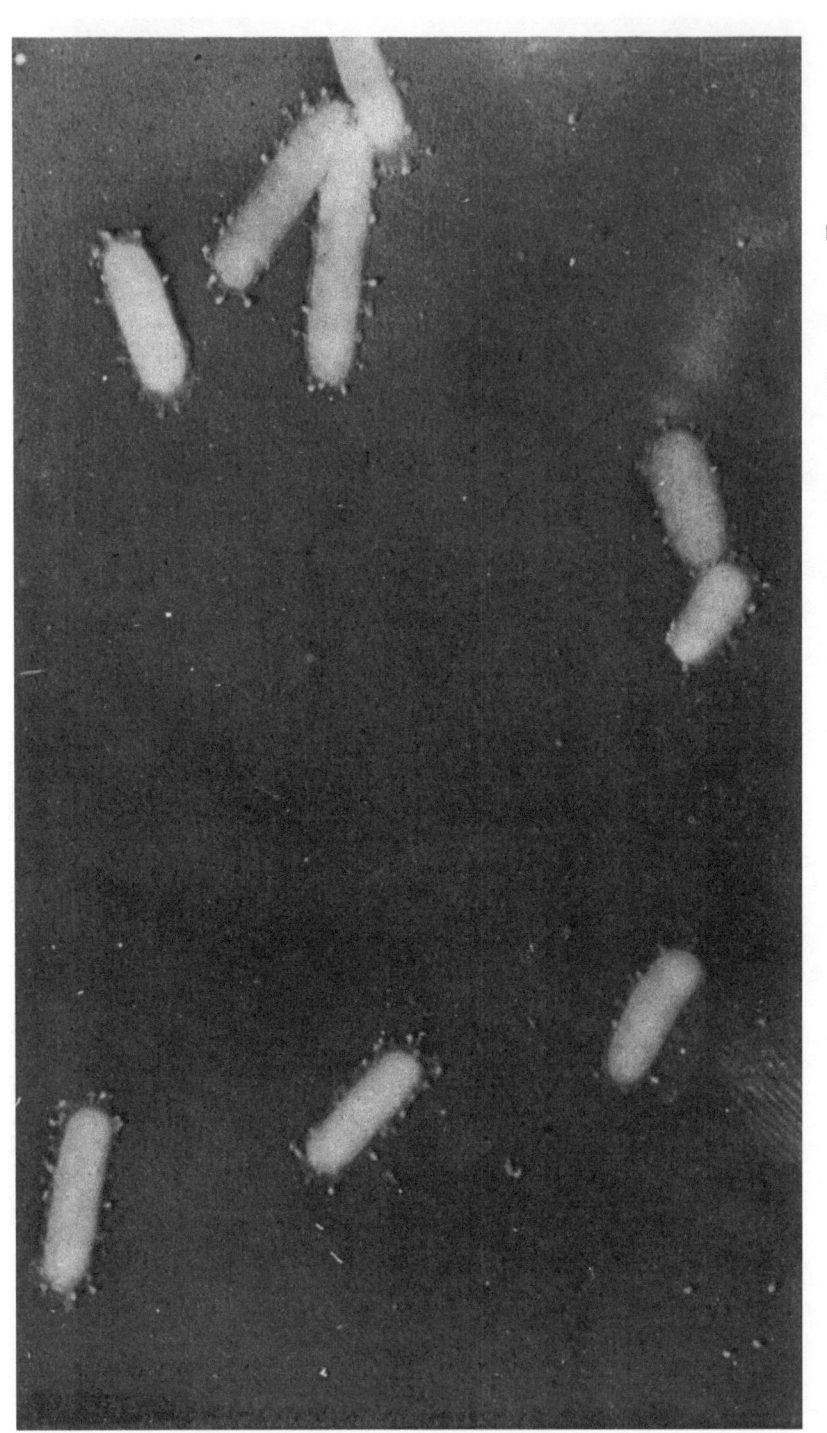

FIGURE 3. AN ELECTRON MICROGRAPH OF HOST BACTERIA WHICH HAD BEEN EXPOSED TO T4 IN THE PRESENCE OF ADDED L-TRYPTOPHANE

Many virus particles have been activated by the tryptophane and can be seen adsorbed to the host cells. EMG 216c.

ml. and then added to host cells in a large volume of ammonium-lactate medium, a sizable fraction of virus is adsorbed, even though the concentration of tryptophan in this adsorption mixture may be 0.02 microgram per ml. On the other hand, the addition of such minute amounts of tryptophan to a mixture of T_4 and host cells induces little, if any, adsorption of virus. That the adsorption process here requires some time for its consummation is indicated by the fact that T_4 with cofactor is not adsorbed on host cells in a violently stirred medium; the two seem to be ripped apart by the shearing forces in the liquid before a firm bond can be formed. Give them a few seconds to form such a bond and they are not pulled apart (unpublished results of the author).

The reaction between virus and cofactor seems (13) to be reversible, for on dilution of an activation mixture of virus and tryptophan, the virus loses its adsorbability at a measurable rate but can be reactivated by the addition of more cofactor.

Another condition which affects the percentage of virus activated by a given concentration of tryptophan is the pH, the optimum for activation being around 7.5. Similarly, temperature affects the activation reaction. At 37° the activation seems to be a maximum, while at 0° very little of the virus in the deficient stocks is activated even by 20 micrograms of tryptophan per ml.

All along I had been worrying about the behavior of those stocks of T_4 and T_6 which readily formed plaques on the pure ammonium-lactate medium at 37°. Indeed, all our stocks contained more or less virus of this type, and when their plaques were picked and tested they were found (14) to consist almost entirely of mutants of the nondeficient type. Nevertheless, their rates of adsorption on host cells were found to be low unless a cofactor like L-tryptophan was added to the medium. We could only hazard the guess that at 37° they acquired cofactor from the bacterial metabolism. The observation that low temperatures increased the cofactor requirements suggested a method for testing this possibility, since at a low temperature one might expect the virus to require higher cofactor concentrations for activation and hence to have difficulty in being adsorbed on the host. It turned out (15) that these strains were indeed inefficient in forming plaques on the minimal medium at 15° C. As was to be expected, the addition of tryptophan to the medium restored to unity their plaque-forming efficiency at 15° C.

Putting these observation in other terms, we may state that at 37° the cells are sensitive to these strains because they liberate enough cofactor into the medium to activate the virus. At 15° the amount of cofactor released by the cells is insufficient for activation, and as a result the cells are resistant to the virus. Here the sensitivity or resistance of a cell to the virus depends in a most striking fashion on the metabolism of the host.

A complementary basis for resistance has recently been uncovered by Delbrück (16) in a special strain of T_4 whose activation is blocked by traces of indole. Since cells of *E. coli* break tryptophan down to indole, under certain conditions their metabolism can create situations in which they are resistant to Delbrück's strain of T_4.

To see whether similar cofactor relationships might not exist between the other viruses, T_1, T_2, etc., and their bacterial hosts, their efficiencies of plaque formation were tested at 15° on the ammonium lactate agar. Two of our stocks, T_1 and T_7, turned out to have low efficiencies of plaque formation at the lower temperature. That of T_7 was increased by the addition of amino acids—leucine, isoleucine, norleucine, or methionine. We do not yet know whether these new cofactors influence the adsorption of T_7 on its host (15), or whether they are required in the development of the T_7-host complex to produce and liberate this virus.

The original concept of the adsorption of a virus on its host involved the steric fitting of complementary surface structures in a manner analogous to that postulated for the antigen-antibody reaction. It now would appear that other factors, possibly involving enzymes, may play a role in virus adsorption.

As far as I know, this is the only known case in which chemically defined compounds promote the specific combination between two distinct biological entities (if we omit from discussion substances like musk, which, acting through the olfactory organs and higher nerve centers, attract one animal to another). In the microscopic world the opsonins, in promoting phagocytosis of bacteria, come closest to performing a function like that of the adsorption cofactors. The opsonins are antibodies, (proteins), either specific or nonspecific. They ap-

ACTIVATION BY ADSORPTION COFACTORS

parently cover the bacterium, giving it a surface or electrical charge which is acceptable to the phagocyte.

It is not impossible that the virus cofactors have such an effect but one might suppose that many types of substances could affect the charge or surface of the virus particle. Since the cofactor's specificity resides in the L-α-amino-acid group one might suppose that this group is involved in an important way. Perhaps the adsorption of virus on the host cell involves the synthesis of some specific peptide bridges between the two in which some cofactor must be incorporated, and in order to be incorporated, must be held in a special position on the virus at the time of collision between virus and host cell.

We now know (17) that in the lag phase, before they can multiply on a minimal medium, bacteria must synthesize and liberate to the medium certain essential substances in concentrations sufficient for their growth. It thus seems possible that other substances supplied to the medium by the bacterial metabolism may be required by T_4 for its adsorption, but that tryptophan is the one whose concentration is critically low, and therefore the one whose effect is most easily detected. We thus see the adsorption of virus being regulated not only by the properties of the host cell per se but involving as well the *environment* the host creates for itself in growth. In this sense a fluid containing growing bacteria is analogous to the intercellular fluids of a multicellular organism.

With regard to the action of viruses in higher organisms it is probably generally recognized that different tissues in the body have different metabolic patterns. These are brought out most strikingly by the different secretions of various glands and by the localization of characteristic pigments in different tissues. Thus the tropisms of different viruses may be regulated by the varied metabolic patterns of the groups of cells which make up the animal. It seems not unreasonable to suppose that they render themselves susceptible to a virus attack by the secretion of characteristic virus-activating substances or cofactors.

It also seems possible that a virus which normally produces a mild infection may acquire an increased virulence through association with a type of cell which, though foreign to the body, provides it with a cofactor for adsorption or multiplication. The association of *Hem-*

ophilus influenzae suis and the virus of swine influenza as investigated by Shope is brought to mind. Either agent alone produces only a mild infection, but together they are highly virulent. The bacterium itself may liberate virus cofactor or it may induce the host's cells to do so and so increase the virus pathogenicity.

The relation of virulence to the nutritional state of the host may have a cofactor explanation. Thus the observation (18) that the Lansing strain of poliomyelitis is less virulent to mice kept on a diet low in tryptophan or vitamin B_1 than to mice on an adequate diet is analogous to my initial observation that T_4 is inefficient in forming plaques on its host in a deficient medium. Because of the complex and self-regulating nature of the intercellular fluids in higher animals it may be difficult to show whether the lack of tryptophan or B_1 reduces the adsorbability of the virus particles on susceptible cells or affects some other phase of the interaction between the two.

The process of adsorption seems to be the optimum point at which to interrupt the life cycle of a virus. As I have already pointed out, once a virus particle is adsorbed on the host cell, far-reaching changes may be wrought in the cell's economy and the cell lost to the animal. In chemotherapy we should therefore attempt to prevent the virus from spreading to uninfected cells. The cofactor phenomenon points to a *rationale* for the chemotherapy of virus diseases. If the cofactors for some animal virus can be discovered, one will naturally search for analogues which, acting like indole or the pyridylalanines, will inhibit virus activity without affecting the otherwise susceptible host cell.

SUMMARY

Because of the precision and ease of experimentation, the bacterial viruses provide an ideal material for investigations of certain basic properties of viruses. Alone the virus particles seem inert, but once adsorbed on the host cell, they divert its synthetic processes to virus production. Unrelated strains cannot both multiply within the same cell but related strains, infecting the same host cell, produce hybrid types which combine the genic properties of the infecting strains.

It has been shown that some of these viruses remain indifferent to their host cells unless supplied with certain amino-acids of the natur-

TABLE 1
Compounds which Promote the Activity of T_4 and T_6 on Their Host in Minimal Medium

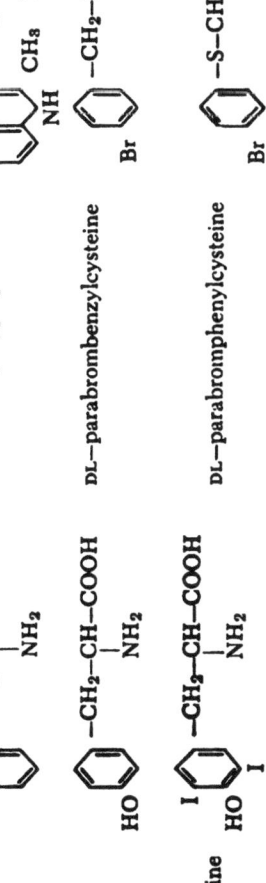
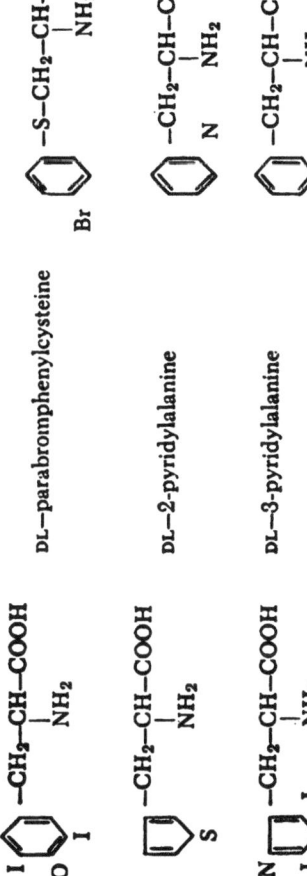

ally occurring L configuration called cofactors. Then they are readily adsorbed to initiate the reaction chains by which the cell is converted to virus production.

Certain virus strains acquire cofactors from the uninfected cell, which thus, by the very nature of its own metabolism, renders itself susceptible to the virus attack.

These phenomena suggest that cofactor mechanisms may play a role in the behavior of animal viruses, and provide a *rationale* for the chemotherapy of virus diseases.

REFERENCES

1. Demerec, M., and U. Fano, Bacteriophage-resistant mutants in *Escherichia coli*, *Genetics*, 1945, 30:119. Cf. p. 250.
2. Anderson, T. F., Morphological and chemical relationships in viruses and bacteriophages, *Cold Spring Harbor Symp. Quant. Biol.*, 1946, 11:1.
3. Delbrück, M., The bacteriophages, *Biol. Rev.*, 1946, 9:332.
4. Delbrück, M., Experiments with bacterial viruses (bacteriophages), *Harvey Lecture Series*, 1946, 41:161. Pp. 216, 253, 255.
5. Henle, W., G. Henle, and E. B. Rosenberg, The demonstration of one-step growth curves of influenza viruses through the blocking effect of irradiated virus on further infection, *J. Exp. Med.*, 1947, 86:423.
6. Cohen, S. S., and T. F. Anderson, Chemical studies on host-virus interactions, I: The effect of bacteriophage adsorption on the multiplication of its host, *Escherichia coli* B, with an appendix giving some data on the composition of the bacteriophage T 2, *J. Exp. Med.*, 1946, 84:511.
7. Monod, J., and E. Wollman, Inhibition of enzymic adaptation in *Escherichia coli*, affected by a bacteriophage, *C. R. Acad. Sci.*, Paris, 1947, 224:417.
8. Hershey, A. D., Spontaneous mutations in bacterial viruses, *Cold Spring Harbor Symp. Quant. Biol.*, 1946, 11:67. P. 250.
9. Hershey, A. D., and R. Rotman, Linkage among genes controlling inhibition of lysis in a bacterial virus, *Proc. Nat. Acad. Sci.*, 1948, 34:89.
10. Anderson, T. F., The growth of T2 virus on ultraviolet-killed host cells, *J. Bact.*, 1948, 56:403.
11. Anderson, T. F., The role of tryptophan in the adsorption of two bacterial viruses on their host *E. coli.*, *J. Cell. & Comp. Physiol.* 1945, 25:17.
12. Anderson, T. F., The activity of a bacteriostatic substance in the reaction between bacterial virus and host, *Science*, 1945, 101:565.
13. Anderson, T. F., The activation of the bacterial virus T4 by L-tryptophan, *J. Bact.*, 1948, 55:637.
14. Anderson, T. F., The inheritance of requirements for adsorption cofactors in the bacterial virus T4, *J. Bact.*, 1948, 55:651.
15. Anderson, T. F., The influence of temperature and nutrients on plaque

formation by bacteriophages active on Escherichia coli, strain B, *J. Bact.*, 1948, 55:659.
16. Delbrück, M., Biochemical mutants of bacterial viruses, *J. Bact.*, 1948, 56:1.
17. Hinshelwood, C. N., *The Chemical Kinetics of the Bacterial Cell* (New York, 1946).
18. Jones, J. H., C. Foster, W. Henle, and D. Alexander, Dietary deficiencies and poliomyelitis, effects of low protein and of low tryptophan diets on the response of mice to the Lansing strain of poliomyelitis virus, *Arch. Biochem.*, 1946, 11:481.

Chapter 6

THE ELECTRON MICROSCOPIC STUDY OF VIRUS GROWTH

By RALPH W. G. WYCKOFF, *Laboratory of Physical Biology, Experimental Biology and Medicine Institute, National Institutes of Health*

PHYSICAL and physico-chemical techniques introduced over the last twenty years have profoundly altered, and enlarged, our knowledge of viruses. Thus the development of ultracentrifugation, especially of ultracentrifuges capable of handling large volumes, has enabled us to prepare viruses in the pure and unaltered state that is a necessary preliminary to their precise characterization and to the determination of their chemical composition. The electron microscope in its turn makes it possible to see with what we are dealing, to recognize the elementary particles of those viruses that can be obtained in a sufficiently pure condition, and hence to deal with them with the same assurance that the optical microscope gave to the handling of bacteria and other microorganisms.

As has long been known, viruses, as the submicroscopic causative agents of infectious disease in man and other animals, in plants, and in bacteria, have particle sizes that range in a more or less unbroken series from the lower limit of optical microscopic vision down to about $10m\mu$, a diameter that is considerably smaller than that of many large protein molecules. In the ten years during which electron microscopes have been available the elementary particles of a considerable number of these viruses have been identified and measured. The resulting ability to recognize the particles of a virus as they occur in nature permits a direct experimental approach to a problem that must be met if their fundamental nature is to be understood; namely, how they grow and multiply, or are multiplied, within the living cells that are their hosts. The fact that viruses have dimensions comparable with those of the bigger protein molecules means that in attacking this problem one inevitably sees at the same time into the molecular fine structure of cellular protoplasm and thus acquires a

ELECTRON MICROSCOPIC STUDY OF VIRUS GROWTH 63

new insight into the essential details of the living process. The electron micrographs that follow illustrate the kind of information that can now be gained concerning these questions.

The most extensively studied large animal viruses have been those responsible for either the pox or the psittacosis groups of disease. The original photographs of Greene, Smadel, and Anderson brought out the brick-like aspect of the pox elementary bodies (1). Later work demonstrates a complex organization that expresses itself in a detailed fine structure and an enclosing membrane analogous to that seen in bacteria and other micro-organisms. Psittacosis bodies are spheres of similar complexity that ordinarily collapse under the evacuation incidental to electron microscopy and leave behind their surrounding membranes. It is not yet known how the pox elementary bodies develop, but in preparations of the psittacosis viruses one often sees larger objects; these are groups of several smaller spheres which may be partially matured forms of the virus (Fig. 1).

Until recently the particles of no correspondingly big plant virus have been recognized, largely because such large viruses are to be expected among insect-transmitted infections especially hard to study under laboratory conditions. Examination of concentrations of the infectious principle of one of the more stable of these, that causing potato yellow dwarf, however, shows its probable elementary particle as a fragile submicroscopic bacillary form (2).

The best studied middle-sized virus is that responsible for influenza. Its mature forms are spheres whose variable diameters are distributed in size about a mean. In preparations made from freshly isolated strains there are also present many rods of the same diameter, frequently terminated by spheres; and there is accumulating evidence that they too are forms, perhaps immature, of the influenza virus (Fig. 2).

The small animal viruses thus far recognized, such as those of the Shope papilloma virus and of the encephalomyelitises as photographed by Beard and his co-workers, have all had spherical elementary bodies that did not show an evident fine structure; nothing is yet known of how their particles are produced. The same thing can be said of the virus of poliomyelitis, though the recognition of its particles, as of the particles of any virus derived from nervous tissue, cannot perhaps be considered as entirely certain. The particles of the small plant

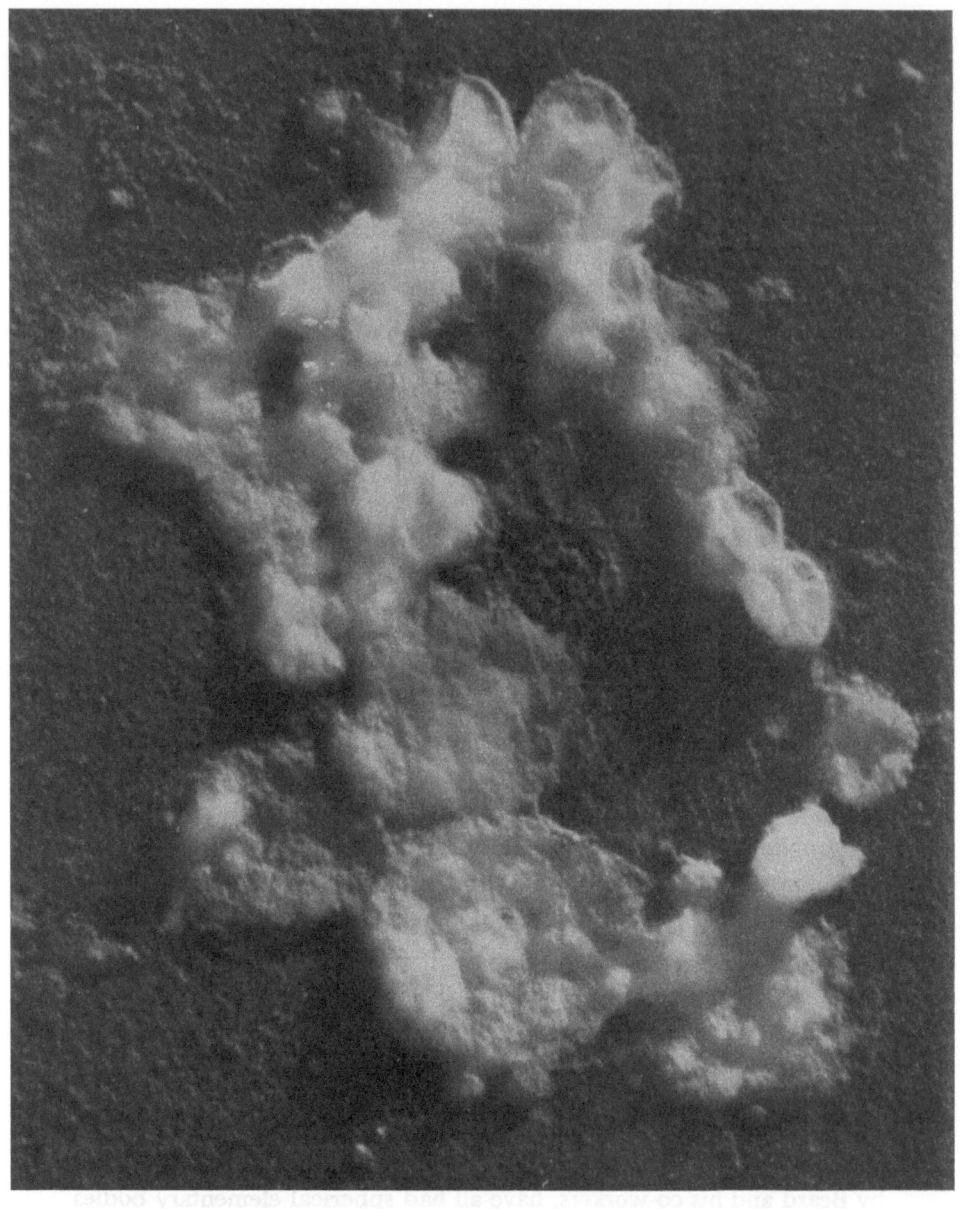

FIGURE 1. AN ELECTRON MICROGRAPH OF A CENTRIFUGALLY PURIFIED SUSPENSION FROM ALLANTOIC FLUID OF CHICK EMBRYO INFECTED WITH A STRAIN OF PSITTACOSIS VIRUS

Chromium shadowing. The elementary bodies of the virus are the collapsed spheres that occur in chains at the left of the group. The larger flat circular objects at the right, containing smaller flattened spheres, may be developing forms. Magnification = × 34,000.

viruses thus far investigated, except those belonging to the tobacco mosaic and potato X groups, also are small and uniformly sized spheres. Williams (3) has shown close associations of spheres of the

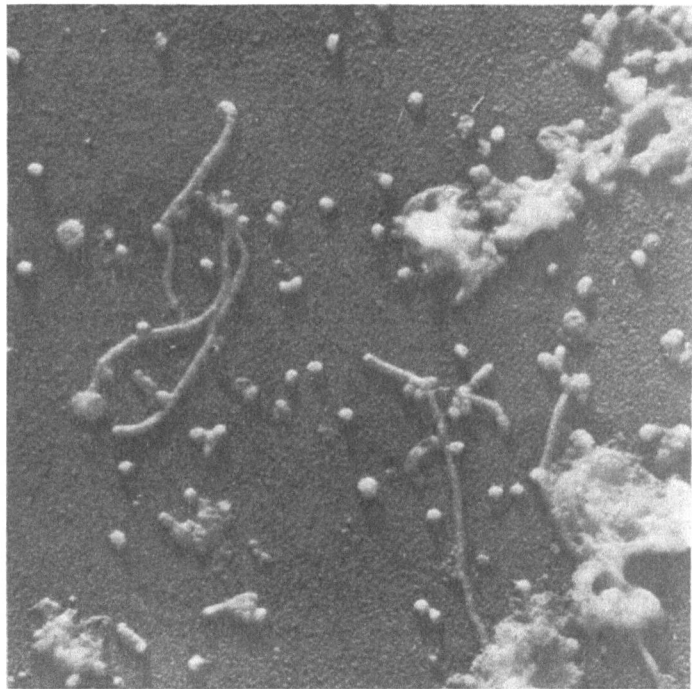

FIGURE 2. TYPICAL FIELD IN AN ELECTRON MICROGRAPH OF AN ULTRACENTRIFUGALLY PURIFIED SUSPENSION FROM FLUID OF CHICK EMBRYOS DISEASED WITH A RECENTLY ISOLATED STRAIN OF TYPE A INFLUENZA VIRUS
The intimate association of filaments with spherical particles is evident. Palladium shadowing. Magnification = × 17,000.

bushy stunt virus which could be interpreted as forms produced by division; nothing else is yet known about the development of any of these virus particles.

In order to gain an adequate understanding of the way particles of any virus develop it is essential to be able to examine them within the cells that are their hosts. Such investigations cannot yet be carried out with the plant viruses we otherwise know most about, because of uncertainties about the cells in which they originate. Most cells that are hosts to animal viruses grow only as tissues. In a few instances, they can be cultivated, as a single cell spreads thin enough for the electron microscope, but usually they must be studied in section. Important progress has been made towards providing sections of the extreme thinness needed for this work, but much remains to be done before fully satisfying studies can be made of sectioned material.

It is much easier to see the internal details in cells that grow as separate individuals. Partly for this reason, bacteria and the bacteriophages that grow at their expense are especially rewarding systems for the study of virus development. Over the last two years renewed electron microscopic investigations have been made of the infection of colon bacilli by the seven strains of bacteriophage designated as T_1 to T_7. The even-numbered of these have sperm-shaped particles whose elongated heads about 60 by 80 mμ in diameter and relatively short straight tails (Fig. 3) make them especially easy to recognize. The odd-numbered bacteriophages have spherical heads and long curved tails. The heads of the different strains range in diameter from about 35 mμ to about 100 mμ; the tails of T_3 and T_7 are so delicate and easily broken off that these strains have hitherto been considered tailless. There are great differences in the rate at which these various bacteriophages cause lysis, and perhaps largely for this reason the accompanying phenomena differ profoundly from strain to strain. The most detailed efforts (4) have thus far been devoted to interpretation of the action of the T_2 (and T_4) and the T_3 strain.

Electron microscopic observations of the phenomena of bacterial lysis have been made, using both solid and liquid cultures. To make preparations from a liquid culture, suspensions of bacteriophage have been mixed with cultures of growing bacteria. After the desired incubation the organisms have been separated by centrifugation, washed with saline and water, and placed on the usual collodion membranes for metal shadowing. Cultures of bacteria infected with bacteriophage growing on solid media have been prepared for electron microscopy by flooding the growing surface with dilute collodion, draining, and allowing the resulting film to harden. Such films, containing embedded within them the top layers of organisms, have then been floated off onto a water surface, washed with water, and mounted on screens for shadowing. The latter technique permits the study of bacteriophage and bacteria in the relative positions they

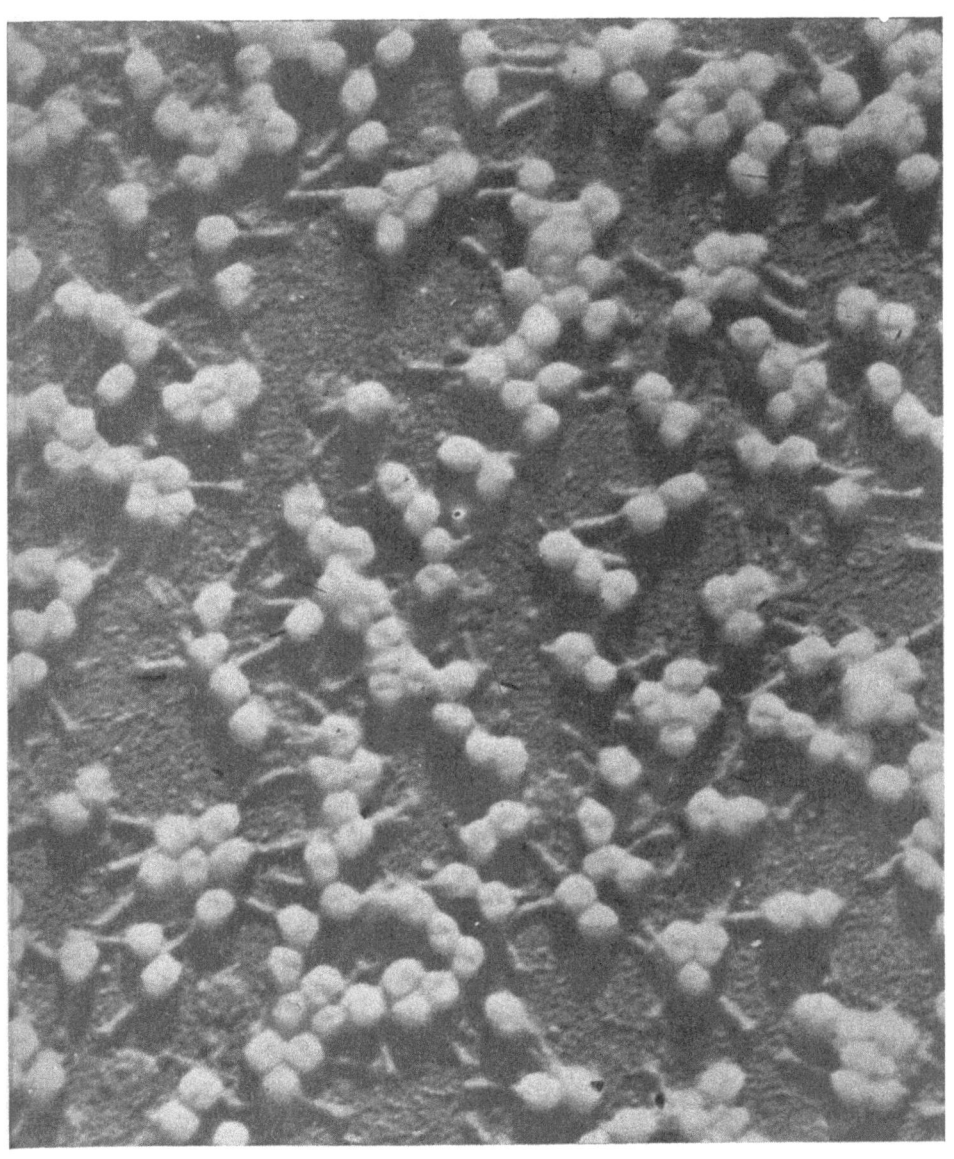

FIGURE 3. A FIELD FROM AN ULTRACENTRIFUGALLY PURIFIED SUSPENSION OF THE T$_4$ BACTERIOPHAGE AGAINST *E. coli*
Palladium shadowing. Magnification = × 85,000.

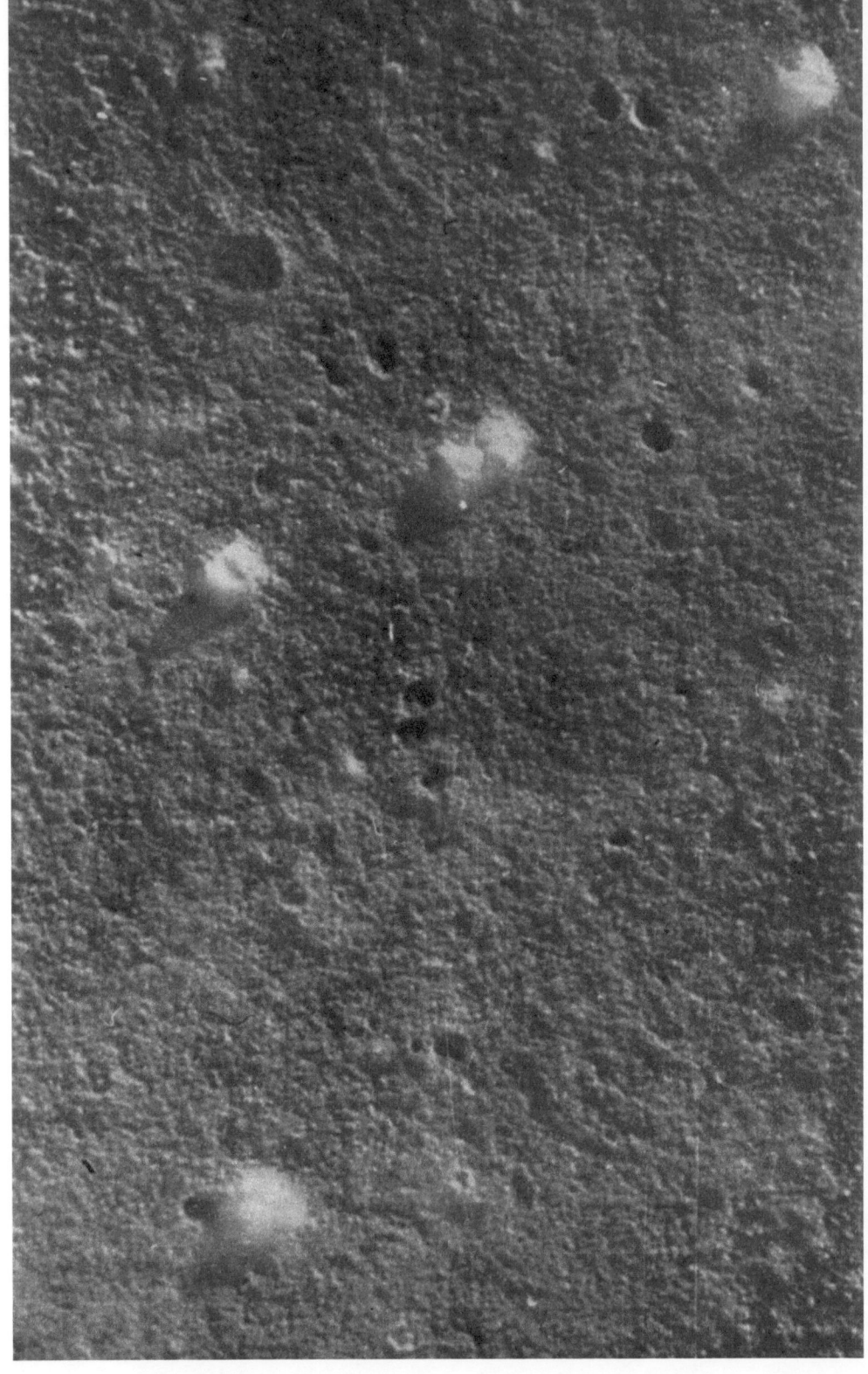

ELECTRON MICROSCOPIC STUDY OF VIRUS GROWTH 69

have during growth, as well as their distribution over various parts of a plaque; it has the disadvantage that the products of bacterial metabolism also are caught in the collodion film, which therefore is not as clean as are preparations made from liquid cultures. For an adequate understanding it is important to study preparations made in both ways.

One of the most striking observations made on lyzed bacteria involves the completeness with which their protoplasm can be converted into particles of bacteriophage. In many cases there has been little left of the original bacterial body after infection with T_4 and T_8 bacteriophages except fragments of membrane and some unused fibrous strands. Especially after infection with T_3, the resulting new bacteriophage particles may be so tightly packed within the confines of the old bacterial cell that they assume a regularity of arrangement which is almost crystalline.

The phenomena of lysis as seen in the electron microscope depend not only on the strain of bacteriophage but also, and strikingly, on the age of the bacterial culture undergoing lysis. When the bacteria of a three- or four-hour-old culture are diseased, the resulting masses of bacteriophage commonly retain the outlines of the cells in which they develop, but with very young and rapidly growing cultures, obtained by several transfers at hourly intervals, different and sometimes more illuminating electron micrographs are obtained. Such bacteria may be lyzed almost immediately after having adsorbed particles of T_2 bacteriophage, and their protoplasm is so fluid that it seems to flow out of the lyzed cell and engulf the invading bacteriophage. Several hundred electron micrographs have now been made of the lysis of such young bacteria with T_2 bacteriophage, and these show numerous steps in the development of new particles from this infection. The engulfed invaders first seem to enlarge to form opaque masses several times larger than the particles themselves (Fig. 4). At first little can be seen of the fine structure within these thick masses, but with longer incubation the embedding protoplasm becomes thinner, and then it is clear that the masses consist of several

---

FIGURE 4. PROTOPLASM FROM PART OF A COLON BACILLUS LYZED THROUGH THE ACTION OF THE T_2 STRAIN OF BACTERIOPHAGE
Palladium shadowing. Magnification = × 60,000.

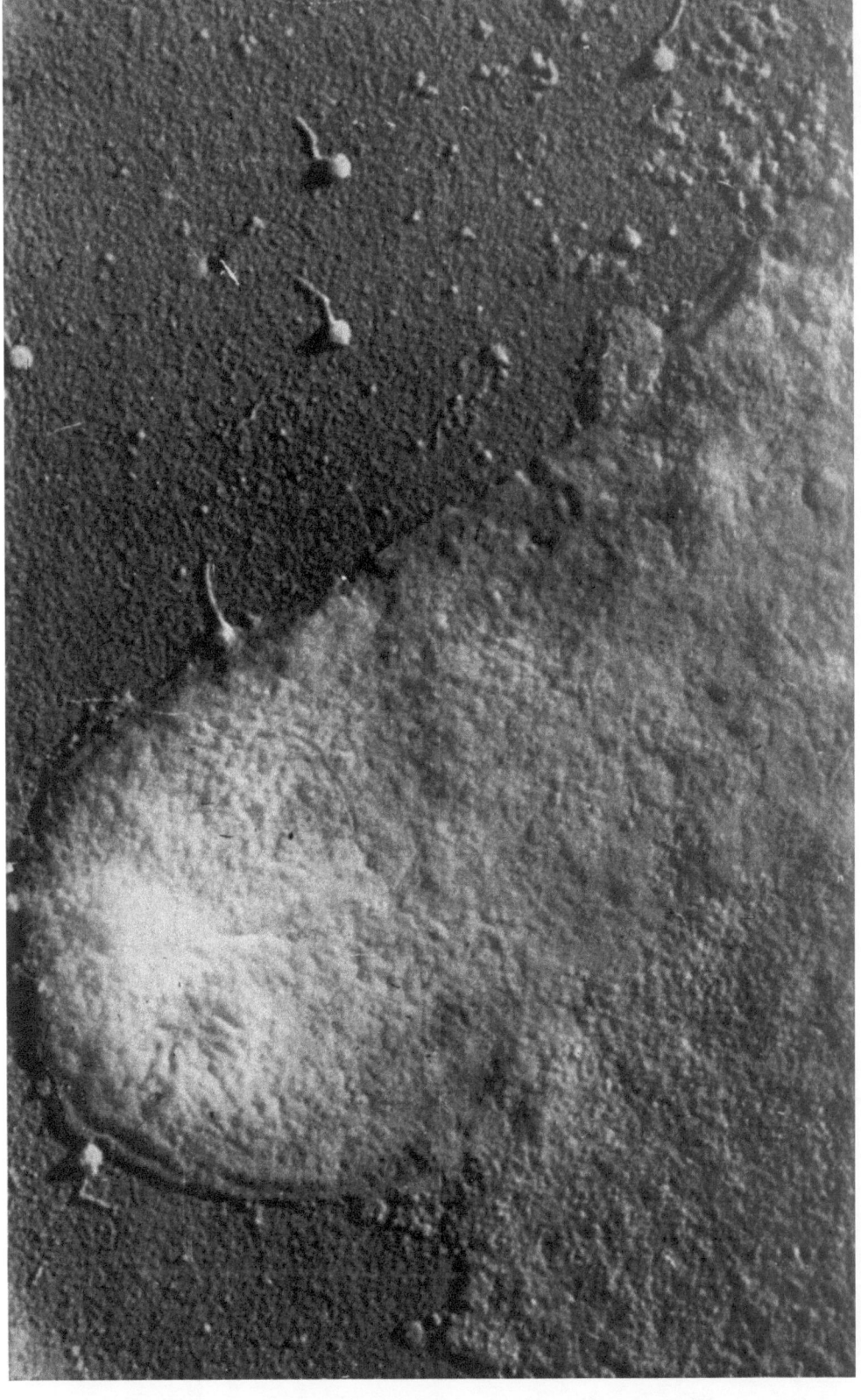

particles similar to but usually somewhat smaller than the mature particles of bacteriophage. The particles in these groups often exhibit short tails, or none at all. After longer incubation the original bacterial protoplasm has almost completely disappeared and the groups are more or less dispersed. At this stage pairs of particles are unusually frequent. It is much harder to interpret what is seen during the growth of bacteriophage in older bacteria that retain their cellular outlines after infection. Nevertheless, many of the photographs obtained of older cells suggest that here too the invading particles serve as centers of bacteriophage proliferation. Such series of electron micrographs have shown the sequence to be expected if this phage is a parasite growing at the expense of the protoplasm of the bacteria it attacks and multiplying by a process analogous to that by which the coccoid bacteria, for instance, reproduce. The experiments with young, actively metabolizing, bacteria indicate that lysis can occur almost immediately after contact between bacteria and bacteriophage; they point to the rather surprising conclusion that multiplication may under such circumstances occur in masses of protoplasm that no longer are contained within intact cells.

Information about the growth of other strains of bacteriophage against *E. coli* and other organisms is still fragmentary, but what is available is compatible with the assumption that they too are self-reproducing. To the degree to which bacteriophages can be considered as typical viruses, these results are evidence for their similarity to micro-organisms.

The bacterial protoplasm seen in these electron micrographs has a surprisingly simple structure. That freed from the very young bacteria has consisted almost entirely of spherical particles of a uniform diameter somewhat less than 10 mμ (Figs. 4, 5). It is these particles that decrease in number as the bacteriophage particles multiply and that therefore seem to provide the substance utilized for their growth. In the protoplasm of older bacteria these spherical particles are

---

FIGURE 5. A STAGE IN THE ATTACK BY T5 PARTICLES OF BACTERIOPHAGE ON A GROUP OF SUSCEPTIBLE COLON BACILLI

The lyzed protoplasm at the right of the photograph is a mass of the same kind of spherical macromolecules as that seen in Figure 4. In this photograph, as in many others, attacking particles all approach a bacterium head-on. Chromium shadowing. Magnification = × 64,000.

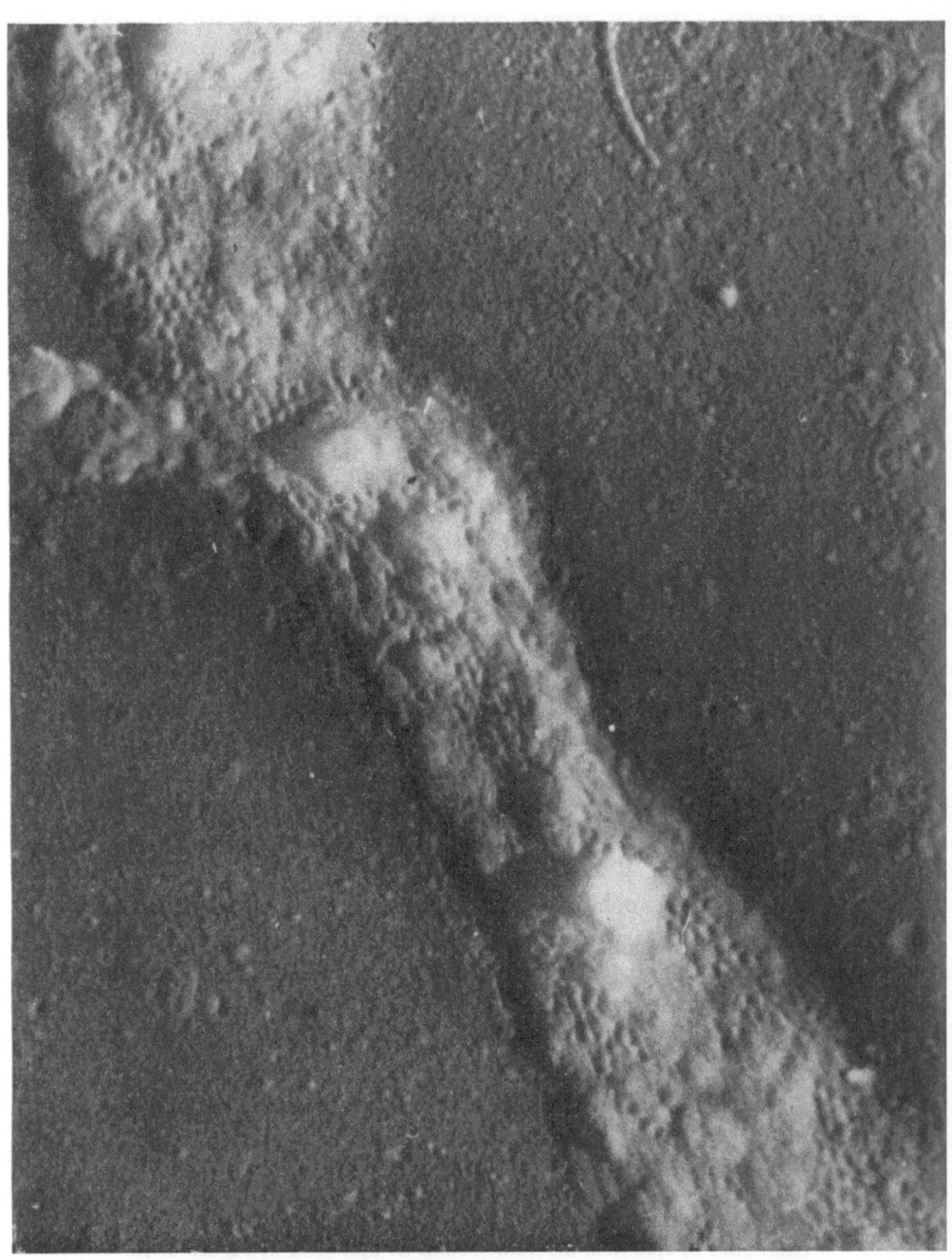

FIGURE 6. PART OF AN OLD COLON BACILLUS AFTER LYSIS BY T7 BACTERIOPHAGE

The framework of fibrous material left behind after bacteriophage multiplication is clearly seen. Chromium shadowing. Magnification = × 45,000.

accompanied by delicate fibrous strands of macromolecular dimensions, which seem to become more numerous as a bacterium ages. This fibrous component seemingly is not utilized by the developing bacteriophage and hence is especially apparent in the residues of lyzed older cells (Fig. 6). The protoplasm of older bacteria gives evidence of becoming more viscous with age, and it is likely that the gelatinous character is to be attributed to this fibrous substrate. It is of course an interesting question whether this protoplasmic fine structure is that of the original intact bacterial cell or is induced by the action of the attacking bacteriophage. This cannot be answered with complete certainty at the present time, but there are important reasons for believing that normal protoplasm has this fine structure. In any event it is obvious that electron microscopic techniques are now in a position to give direct and intimate information about the macromolecular structure of bacterial, and of other, protoplasm. The next few years should see a great increase in our knowledge of this structure, as well as of details of the processes whereby protoplasm is used by viruses for their growth. Working with such virus particles, many of them no bigger than the larger protein molecules but endowed with some at least of the properties of living matter, we cannot avoid at the same time approaching closer to a satisfactory understanding and definition of certain essentials of the living process.

REFERENCES

1. For detailed bibliography see R. W. G. Wyckoff, *J. A. M. A.*, 1948, 136: 1081.
2. Black, L. M., V. M. Mosley, and R. W. G. Wyckoff, *Biochim. Biophys. Acta*, 1948, 2:121.
3. Williams, R. C., 1948 meeting of Electron Microscope Society of America.
4. Wyckoff, R. W. G., *Biochim. Biophys. Acta*, 1948, 2:27, 246; *Nature*, 1948: 162, 649.

Chapter 7

PATHOLOGY AND PATHOGENESIS OF THE CUTANEOUS LESIONS OF VARIOLA, VACCINIA, HERPES SIMPLEX, HERPES ZOSTER, AND VARICELLA

By T. F. McNair Scott, H. Blank, L. L. Coriell, and H. Crouse, *Department of Pediatrics, The Children's Hospital of Philadelphia, and Department of Dermatology and Syphilology and Department of Zoology, School of Medicine, University of Pennsylvania*

The response of the skin to noxious agents follows the general pattern of the body responses, but because of the peculiarities of skin structure, this pattern tends to be modified, and experience is often required before changes seen can be interpreted. Hence, consideration of the pathological changes in the skin is accounted a subspecialty of pathology as a whole.

Since, also, the superficial position of the skin makes it easily accessible for study, an accurate interpretation of the histologic changes that occur in different disease states takes an even more prominent position, perhaps, in the analysis of the pathogenesis of such diseases than does general pathology in the realm of general medicine.

In the field of viral infections, a study of the pathology of certain diseases that affect the skin early demonstrated that peculiar changes occurred regularly and appeared to be specific for the individual disease examined. In general, these peculiar changes took the form of "intracellular bodies" with tinctorial and morphological properties that differed from those of the rest of the involved cell and were not present at all in normal cells. Although many types of cell inclusions are recognized by cytologists as belonging to the normal structure of the cell, it seemed clear that the "inclusion bodies" just referred to were not in this category but were associated in some way with the virus infection.

The application of histochemistry, by means of which the presence of specific chemical elements can be demonstrated in tissue sections by means of certain color reactions, has led to an appreciation of the fact that study of a stained section may reveal information not only of the morphological structure but also of the chemical structure of the tissue examined. Since viruses are intracellular parasites and presumably grow by diverting into virus, in some way, the chemical elements that would normally be synthesized into cell protoplasm, the importance of this viewpoint in the histopathological study of this group of diseases is self-evident. Even the routine hematoxylin and eosin stain with its characteristic coloration of different parts of the cell (1) may be interpreted as indicating in a crude way that the different parts of the cell have different chemical compositions. The deep blue staining, regardless of the type of fixation, of the nuclear chromatin by the hematoxylin, the so-called basophilic reaction, can be associated with the presence of desoxyribose nucleic acid. This is absent from the cytoplasm and from the nucleolus, which take the pink eosin stain, giving rise to the so-called acidophilic or eosinophilic reaction. A similar eosinophilic reaction might also indicate that degeneration had occurred and normal nucleoprotein was absent. Since all viruses appear to contain nucleoprotein and since in all the larger animal viruses so far studied, this appears to be of the desoxyribose nucleic acid type, the application of this kind of interpretation to the study of inclusion bodies has useful implications. Thus, on the basis of a routine section, it may be possible to form a tentative conclusion as to whether the tinctorial characteristics of any inclusion body are compatible with the presence of virus or not. If it stained like the nuclear chromatin and therefore probably contained desoxyribose nucleic acid, it would certainly be more likely to contain actual virus than if it did not.

The application of more specific stains for nucleic acid may help to confirm this opinion. For instance, toluidine blue stain will indicate by a blue color the presence of either type of nucleic acid and at least confirm the presence or absence of nucleoprotein in the structure being considered, while the Feulgen stain (decolorized basic fuchsin) will demonstrate specifically the presence of desoxyribose nucleic acid by being recolored pink. Naturally, no more than a working hypothesis can be based on such findings, which must be correlated with actual evidence of infectivity before definite conclusions can be drawn. However, since considerable weight is placed on staining reactions in the controversy which still exists as to the exact nature of inclusion bodies, it seemed advisable to draw attention to this aspect of histopathology.

Inclusion bodies are of two types: those occurring in the cytoplasm or cytoplasmic, and those occurring in the nucleus, or intranuclear inclusion bodies. The former are characteristic of the variola-vaccinia group of infections, while the latter are similarly characteristic of herpes simplex, zoster, and varicella. There exists a division of opinion as to whether these bodies actually represent virus or are merely evidence of cell alteration or degeneration induced by the presence of the virus, which itself remains invisible. Evidence on this point will be discussed in relation to the individual diseases. However, it seems appropriate, in light of the previous discussion, to comment, on the one hand, on the textbook definitions of the inclusion bodies seen in the diseases discussed in this paper, which are commonly accepted as being the one tinctorial and morphological appearance that characterizes any given inclusion, and, on the other hand, the variation in these appearances that are actually described by the many individual investigators who have studied this problem. This difficulty arises because a textbook definition must almost inevitably refer to something static, while the viral infection of a cell is actually a dynamic affair. An appreciation of this point of view will be an aid in the routine interpretation of sections from virus-infected tissues, since any one section may reveal all stages of the cycle from cell invasion through multiplication to release of virus from the cell, each phase having a different tinctorial and morphological representation, only one of which may correspond to the textbook description. On the other hand, for various reasons, one phase or another may predominate in the section.

With this rather general introduction, I will now turn to a more detailed discussion of the specific problem, but before discussing pathology, I want to remind you briefly of the histology of the normal skin (2) (Fig. 1). The skin is differentiated into two main divisions: the corium, or true skin, and the epidermis. The corium, derived from embryonic mesoderm, is made up largely of connective tissue, and contains blood and lymph vessels, nerve fibers, sweat and sebaceous glands, and hairs. The epidermis, derived from embryonic ectoderm, consists of several super-imposed layers of epithelial cells and is divided for descriptive purposes into named strata according to the morphologic appearance of those cells. The stratum germinativum, or basal layer, consists of a single row of columnar cells adjoining

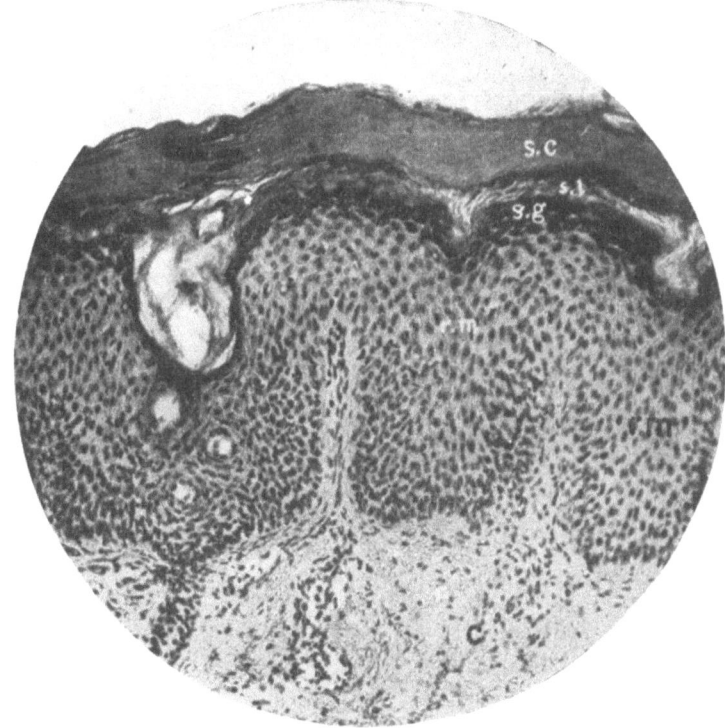

FIGURE 1. NORMAL SKIN
S.c.–Stratum corneum; S.l.–Stratum lucidum; S.g.–Stratum granulosum; R.m.–Rete malpighi; C.–Corium. (From Becker and Obermeyer, *Modern Dermatology and Syphilology*, 2d ed., Philadelphia, J. B. Lippincott, 1947.)

and intimately connected with the corium by a series of interdigitations, called respectively the papillae of the corium and the "rete pegs" of the epidermis. These cells contain most of the pigment granules, when present, and are actively growing. The name "prickle-cell layer" is applied to the four to eight rows of nucleated polyhedral cells which lie immediately external to the basal layer. These are connected with each other by a series of protoplasmic threads called prickles and hence the name. Growth of cells also occurs in this layer. The name "stratum mucosum" or "malpighian layer" is given

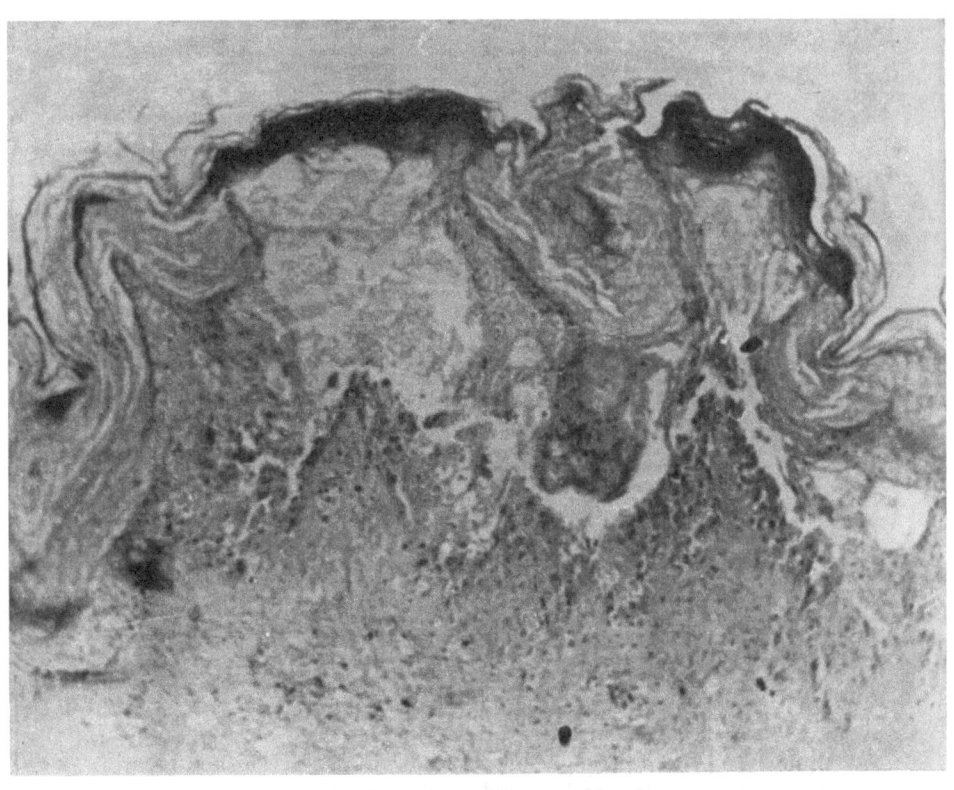

FIGURE 2. VARIOLA. BIOPSY OF HUMAN SKIN SHOWING EDGE OF EARLY VESICLE
Note involvement of epithelium with multilocular vesicle formation and relative absence of involvement of the corium. Hematoxylin and eosin. Magnification = × 80.

PATHOLOGY OF CUTANEOUS LESIONS 79

to the combination of these two innermost layers. Outside this lie several strata of cells undergoing a progression of chemical changes that lead to death and keratinization. These are called, respectively, stratum granulosum, stratum lucidum, and stratum corneum.

The pathology of the diseases under discussion will be considered under two main headings: (1) those characterized by cytoplasmic inclusions and (2) those characterized by intranuclear inclusions.

DISEASES CHARACTERIZED BY CYTOPLASMIC INCLUSIONS

The over-all pathologic picture is very much the same for all three diseases included in this first group—variola major, alastrim (variola minor), and vaccinia. Some observers believe distinguishing details can be observed which differentiate alastrim, or variola minor, from variola major, and these will be mentioned in due course. Torres' (3) description of alastrim in the monkey follows, and, as you can see by the illustrations of human variola major (from Dr. Downie of Liverpool, England), a common description fits both (4) (Figs. 2–4).

Proliferation of the prickle-cell layer occurs early, and in these proliferated cells large numbers of cytoplasmic inclusions can be seen. The nuclei enlarge and small vacuoles appear in the cytoplasm. Following this evidence of early intracellular edema, intercellular edema appears. In the affected cells, particularly those of the upper layers of the thickened stratum mucosum, the vacuoles enlarge and become confluent, distending the cell membrane, which finally breaks down; by coalescence with neighboring, similarly affected cells, small vesicles and, later, large vesicles develop. It is the presence of a large number of closely packed, small vesicles that gives the early lesions of smallpox their firm, shotty feel, and multilocular character. The proliferating epithelial cells force the cuto-epithelial line below the normal level, compressing and finally obliterating the papillary eminences. This epidermal reaction is succeeded by a dilatation of blood and lymph vessels and an accompanying inflammatory cell exudate in the corium. As the disease progresses, the vesicles become larger and become filled with white cells and tissue debris. The floor and sides of a fully formed vesicle are formed of the remaining cells of the malpighian layer, which show edema to a somewhat lesser extent, giving rise to the characteristic so-called "ballooning degen-

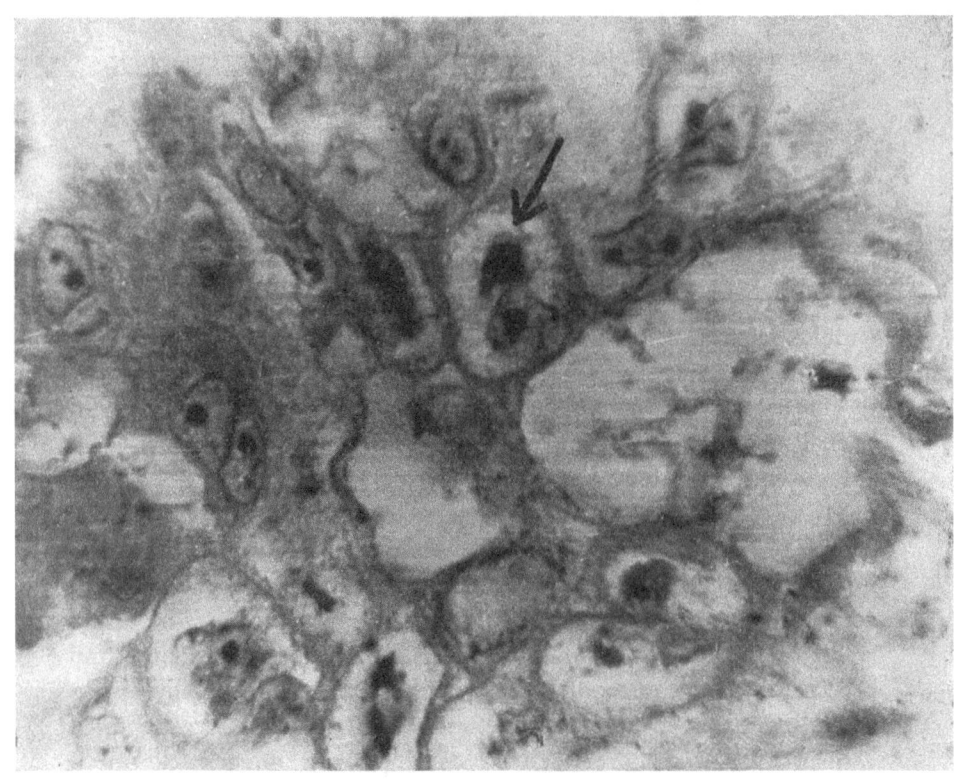

FIGURE 3. VARIOLA. BIOPSY OF HUMAN SKIN SHOWING TREMENDOUS INTRACELLULAR EDEMA WITH DESTRUCTION OF CELL BOUNDARIES (EARLY STAGE OF MULTILOCULAR VESICLE FORMATION)
Note also well-marked, dense, basophilic cystoplasmic inclusion body (Guarnieri body). Hematoxylin and eosin. Magnification = × 900.

eration"; the roof is formed of the cells of the stratum granulosum and outer layers. In alastrim the basilar layer is little, if any, involved, whereas in variola and vaccinia, all the layers appear involved, and the floor of the vesicle is usually formed by the naked corium in which actual necrosis has occurred. This explains the typical scarring that occurs after smallpox and vaccinia, but which is rare in alastrim.

Other diagnostic differences have been claimed between alastrim and variola major, chiefly on the basis of the morphological and tinctorial characteristics of the cytoplasmic inclusion bodies seen in the two diseases; those in alastrim being described as more basophilic and larger than those in variola (5). There is one characteristic, however, which distinguishes both variola and alastrim from vaccinia, and that is the presence, in the former two diseases, and the absence in the latter, of intranuclear as well as cytoplasmic inclusions. In variola, these are not infrequent in the floor of the vesicle and appear to be rather dense, homogeneous, eosinophilic masses occurring in shrunken nuclei. In alastrim, they are described as occurring much less frequently, while the bodies themselves are less distinct and the nucleus is enlarged rather than shrunken.

Whatever the true explanation of the intranuclear inclusions seen in variola and alastrim—they are, at present, considered evidence of cell degeneration—the cytoplasmic inclusions in these diseases are generally accepted as representing colonies of virus particles. These particles, although first described by Buist (6) in 1886, were rediscovered by Paschen (7) in 1906 and are sometimes referred to as Paschen's bodies. These minute elementary bodies have been shown to be the etiologic agent of the variola-vaccinia group of diseases. Electron micrography has improved our knowledge of these bodies and has confirmed strikingly the conclusions reached by visual study, that the inclusion bodies are actually colonies of these minute bodies (8). Although the elementary bodies contain desoxyribose nucleic acid and give a positive Feulgen reaction when tested in bulk (9) in a test tube, the concentration is so low (5.6 percent, according to Hoagland et al [10]) that on the stained smear the individual body is Feulgen-negative, a point which emphasizes the limitations of the histochemical approach. It is interesting to read over the various descriptions of these cytoplasmic inclusions, which were first described by Guarnieri in 1892. He pointed out that they were

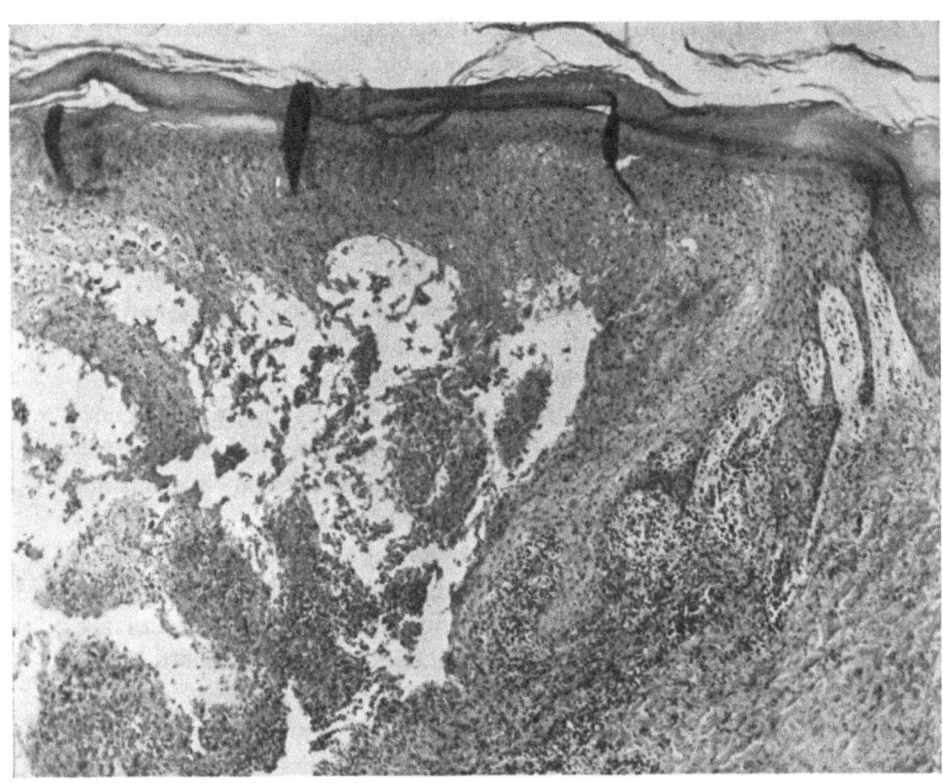

FIGURE 4. VARIOLA. BIOPSY OF HUMAN SKIN SHOWING EDGE OF A LATE VESICLE

Note increased breadth of the malpighian layer of the involved epithelium in contrast to the normal epithelium at extreme edge of picture. Note also the involvement of the corium, necrosis at the base of the vesicle, and diffuse infiltration of inflammatory cells. Hematoxylin and eosin. Magnification = × 44. (Material kindly sent by Prof. A. W. Downie, Liverpool, England.)

strongly stained by safranine and hematoxylin, both basic dyes (11). The description of these bodies in the recent book by van Rooyen and Rhodes (8) is "the large eosinophilic inclusion bodies of variola and vaccinia"; in other words, they stain with an "acid" dye. Nevertheless, from Guarnieri on, differences in size and staining reaction of these bodies have been described repeatedly.

Some of the difficulties in understanding the reason for this diversity have, I think, been removed by the careful analysis by Bland and Robinow (9) of the dynamics of the processes occurring in vaccinia-infected cells. These investigators grew the corneal cells of rabbits in tissue culture, then added purified elementary bodies to the culture, and examined the cells at various times after infection. They were able to point out a series of changes occurring in the infected cells. During the first two hours, they could see that many of the cells contained elementary bodies but that, in addition, small homogeneous bodies had been formed in the cytoplasm. These were considered the earliest stage in the development of a virus colony. During the next ten hours, these bodies grew larger to form large homogeneous bodies. These bodies were replaced by what they called small and medium networks. During this latter phase, elementary bodies were no longer visible in the cells. Finally, large networks developed, which were maximum at twenty-four hours. At this stage, elementary bodies could be seen at the periphery of the cells and appeared to be coming out from the center of the cells.

The following is a description of these same stages in terms of reactions to hematoxylin and eosin, and to Feulgen staining: The elementary bodies tend to be eosinophilic and are Feulgen-negative, as described above. The stages of the small and the large homogeneous body, on the other hand, are strongly basophilic in character and, as might be expected, are Feulgen-positive. It does not seem clear as yet just what this Feulgen-positive material is. The so-called networks are less dense and become progressively more eosinophilic in character and less Feulgen-positive (Fig. 5).

Since, in most sections, cells can be seen in various stages of infection, it is not difficult to understand that diverse morphological and tinctorial properties will be found; perhaps more of one stage or another will predominate, depending on the time after infection and the part of the section studied. In an externally imposed infection,

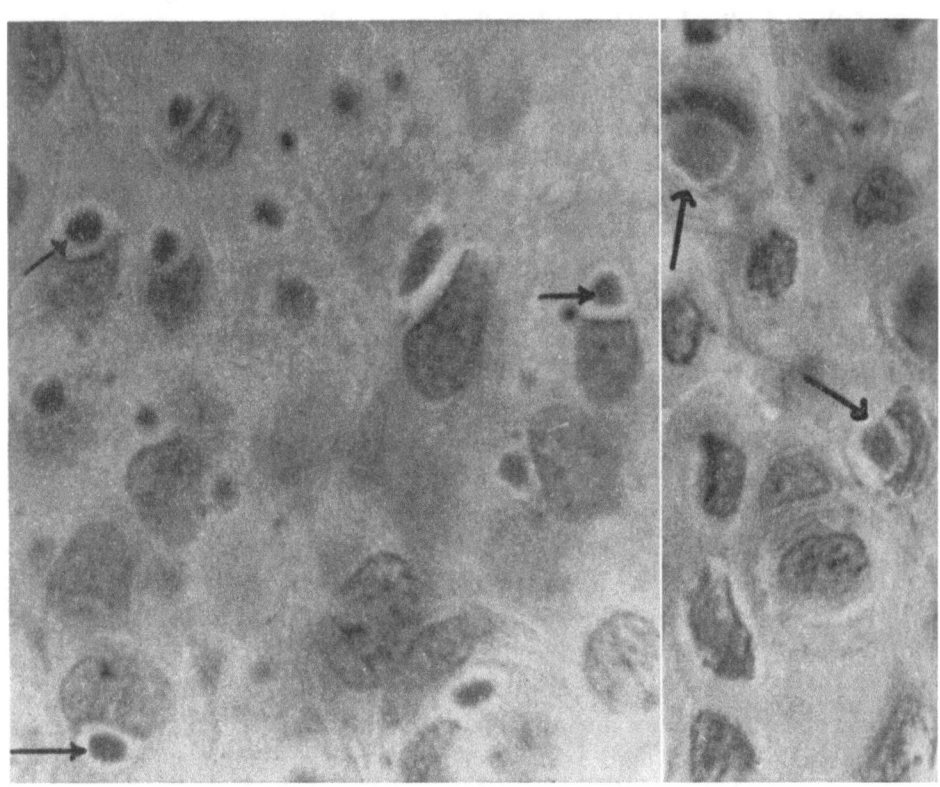

FIGURE 5. VACCINIA. RABBIT'S CORNEA SHOWING (A) MANY SMALL AND MEDIUM, DENSE CYTOPLASMIC INCLUSION BODIES WHICH ARE BASOPHILIC; (B) LARGE, CYTOPLASMIC INCLUSION BODIES, LESS DENSE, AND EOSINOPHILIC
Hematoxylin and eosin. Magnification = × 900.

as on the rabbit's cornea, for instance, when all the cells are presumably infected simultaneously, the inclusions seen will tend to be mainly in the early basophilic phases because, if the tissue is examined at a later stage, most of the diseased cells will have been sloughed off.

DISEASES CHARACTERIZED BY INTRANUCLEAR INCLUSIONS

Of this second group of diseases, consisting of herpes simplex, herpes zoster, and varicella the only one in which the virus is easily recovered and, therefore, available for study is herpes simplex. Elementary bodies have been seen with the electron microscope in herpes zoster and varicella (12) which resemble those of the other pox viruses. In addition, herpes zoster has been transmitted to human skin previously grafted onto the chorio-allantois of the embryonated egg on two occasions (13, 14), but to my knowledge it has not so far been subcultured in this manner. Transmission of both agents has been made in human volunteers (15). In contrast to the variola-vaccinia group of diseases, in which there appears to be either a common agent or a very closely related group of agents for all three diseases, there is no relation between the virus of herpes simplex and those of the other two. The agents of varicella and zoster, however, may be closely related to each other or, possibly, identical. Despite their different nature, each of the three agents produces very similar pathologic changes in the skin, although differences in detail may be revealed by more extensive study.

Goodpasture and Anderson (13), in their one successful transmission of herpes zoster to human skin on egg, describe the development of the lesion. The earliest changes can be seen in the cells of the basal layer of the stratum mucosum or immediately adjacent to it. At this stage there are no inflammatory changes. The cytoplasm and nuclei of the cells become swollen, and the latter contain a large eosinophilic body. As the lesion progresses, more cells become involved and the cells may be enormously swollen. In the most advanced part of the lesion, an inflammatory exudate develops, separating the cells, which, in turn, becomes infiltrated with leucocytes. Giant cells containing eosinophilic inclusions in their nuclei appear in the epithelial exudate. At this point a cellular exudate can be

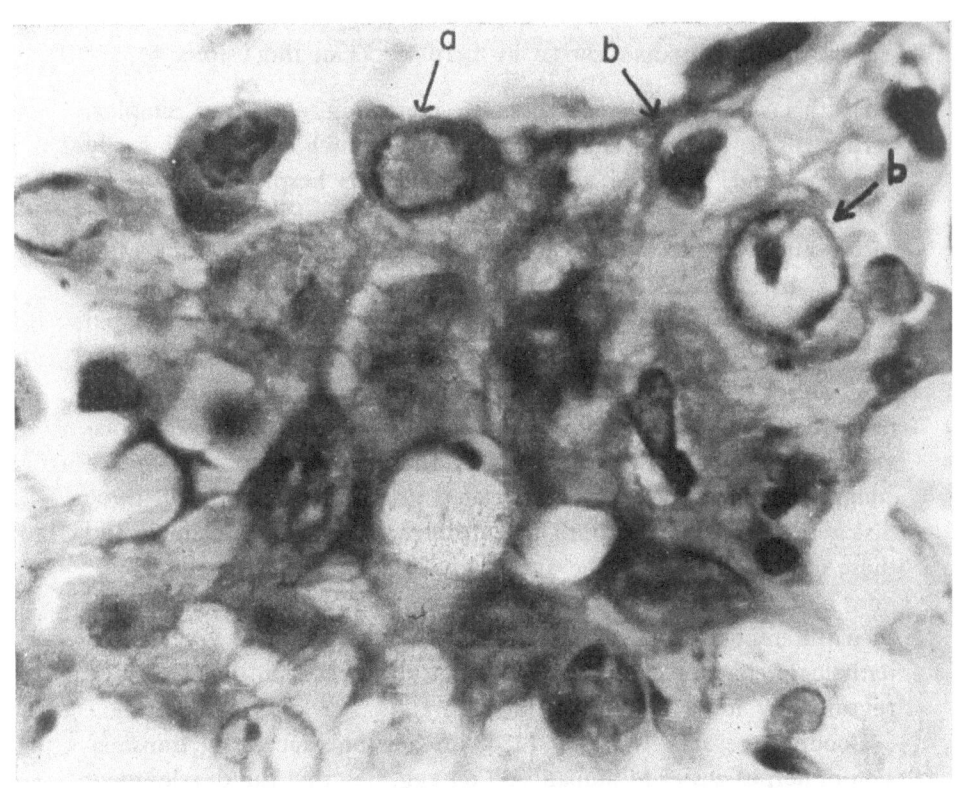

FIGURE 6. HERPES ZOSTER. SHOWING (A) HOMOGENEOUS BASOPHILIC INTRANUCLEAR INCLUSION; (B) CLASSICAL SHRUNKEN, EOSINOPHILIC INCLUSION
Hematoxylin and eosin. Magnification = × 900.

found in the corium. Even in advanced lesions of zoster the cells do not become necrotic. Goodpasture and Anderson point out that herpes simplex infection in similar tissue results in rapid death of cells and ulceration. Furthermore, the intranuclear inclusion bodies in the latter disease become much larger, fill the nucleus, and acquire a basophilic staining reaction. In our experience, this last point is not a good basis of differentiation, since we have seen large basophilic intranuclear inclusions also in herpes zoster (Fig. 6). The significance of this finding will be discussed a little later.

In all three diseases the final lesion, whether on the skin or on the mucous membranes, is a unilocular vesicle. The unilocular characteristics can be recognized even at an early stage and can thus be distinguished from the early multilocular vesicle of the variola-vaccinia group. The difference between the two seems to depend on the different responses of the cells to the two groups of viruses. In the variola-vaccinia group the infection causes tremendous intracellular edema (Fig. 3), so that the fluid collects within the cells as previously described, and there is only a moderate amount of intercellular edema at first. In the herpes group, although there is some intracellular edema as evidenced by the ballooned cells, and some distension and breakdown of cells, the most striking feature is an early and extensive outpouring of fluid between the cells. This starts deep in the malpighian layer and, rapidly separating the cells of this layer, forces some of them to the surface, so that the roof of the single vesicle is composed of malpighian layer (prickle) cells, as well as those of the more external layers (Fig. 7). The walls and floor consist of the remaining cells of the malpighian layer, which are undergoing ballooning degeneration. Sometimes the floor is comprised of the naked papillae of the corium, which are infiltrated with inflammatory cells but which are rarely necrotic. Scarring, therefore, seldom results from these lesions. The exudate consists of an albuminous fluid containing necrotic cell debris, leucocytes, and shed, infected epithelial cells, including the so-called "virus giant cells." There is always an inflammatory reaction in the corium, with dilated blood vessels and cellular exudate (Fig. 8).

In the very early mucous membrane lesions of herpes simplex, actual vesicles can be observed, but usually by the time they come to examination, maceration has resulted in a loss of the fluid and a

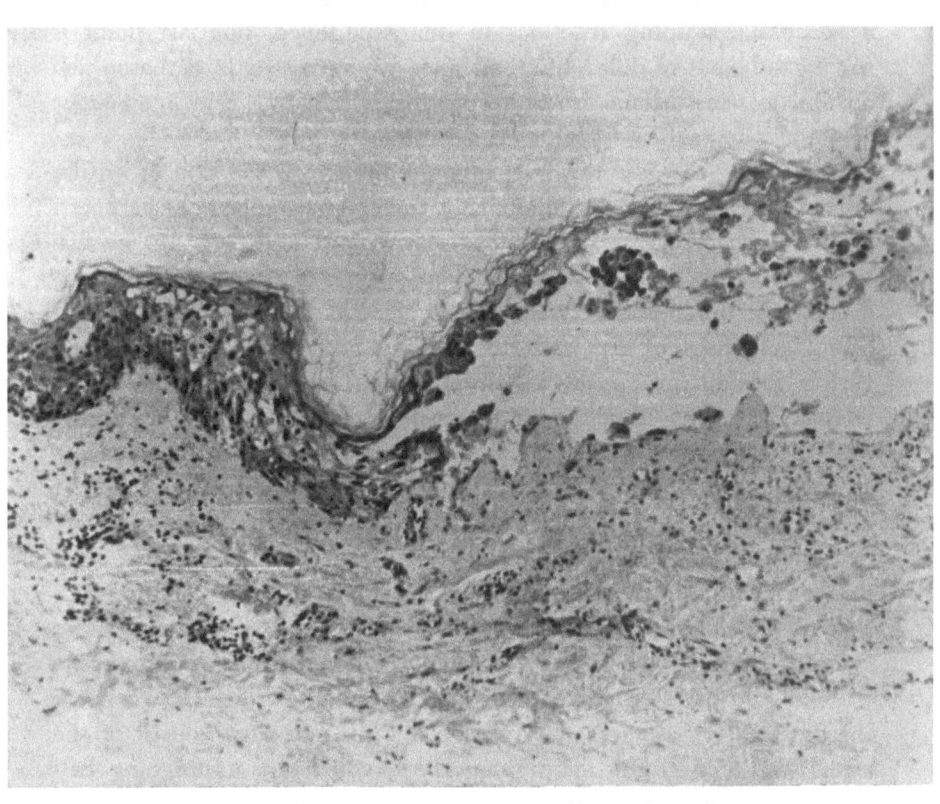

FIGURE 7. VARICELLA. BIOPSY OF HUMAN SKIN SHOWING EDGE OF VESICLE

Note that the split occurs deep in the malpighian layer, so that some of the outer prickle cells help to form the roof of the vesicle. Hematoxylin and eosin. Magnification = × 80.

PATHOLOGY OF CUTANEOUS LESIONS 89

collapse of the roof cells which appear swollen and edematous. These form the white plaque-like lesions so frequently noted clinically. In section, instead of a tense vesicle filled with fluid, a collapsed vesicle is seen, with the cavity filled with cells and fibrin. Otherwise the pictures are identical (Fig. 9).

One of the many problems that arise in the study of herpes is in regard to the exact type of epidermal cells infected by the virus. A biopsy study of a recurrent lesion on the skin of a Negro revealed that the inclusion bodies were confined almost entirely to the pigment-carrying cells; that is to say, the cells of the basal layer (Fig. 10). The same is true for herpes zoster.

As with the previous group, I want now to consider in more detail the inclusion bodies found in this group. The same problem presents itself as in the previous section, but the answer is even less clearly defined. There still exists a considerable difference of opinion between those who, accepting the opinion of Lipschütz (16), who first described these bodies, believe that they represent the virus itself and are in the same category as the Guarnieri body, and those who believe they are merely evidence of cell degeneration. Rivers (17), in his chapter in a recent book on viral and rickettsial diseases, gives the commonly accepted definition of an intranuclear inclusion body, namely, that "it is usually an acidophilic mass occupying most of the nuclear area and is surrounded by a clear zone or halo; the basophilic chromatin of the nucleus marginates on the nuclear membrane." He then goes on to say that although evidence is lacking that virus is present in such nuclei, there is no intrinsic reason why virus should not be there. Some evidence of the infectivity of intranuclear inclusion bodies was produced in 1935 by Baumgartner (18), who isolated the inclusions by microdissection from herpes-infected rabbits' corneae between twenty and thirty hours after inoculation, and reported successful infection of the scarified corneae of other rabbits on two occasions with the washed isolated inclusions, while the washings themselves were negative. This evidence is indeed meager, but it is suggestive and worthy of consideration when the problem is approached from a purely histological standpoint. In reviewing the literature on herpes simplex inclusions, one is again struck by the fallacy of making a single definition of the morphology and staining properties of these inclusions. In 1925, Goodpasture (19)

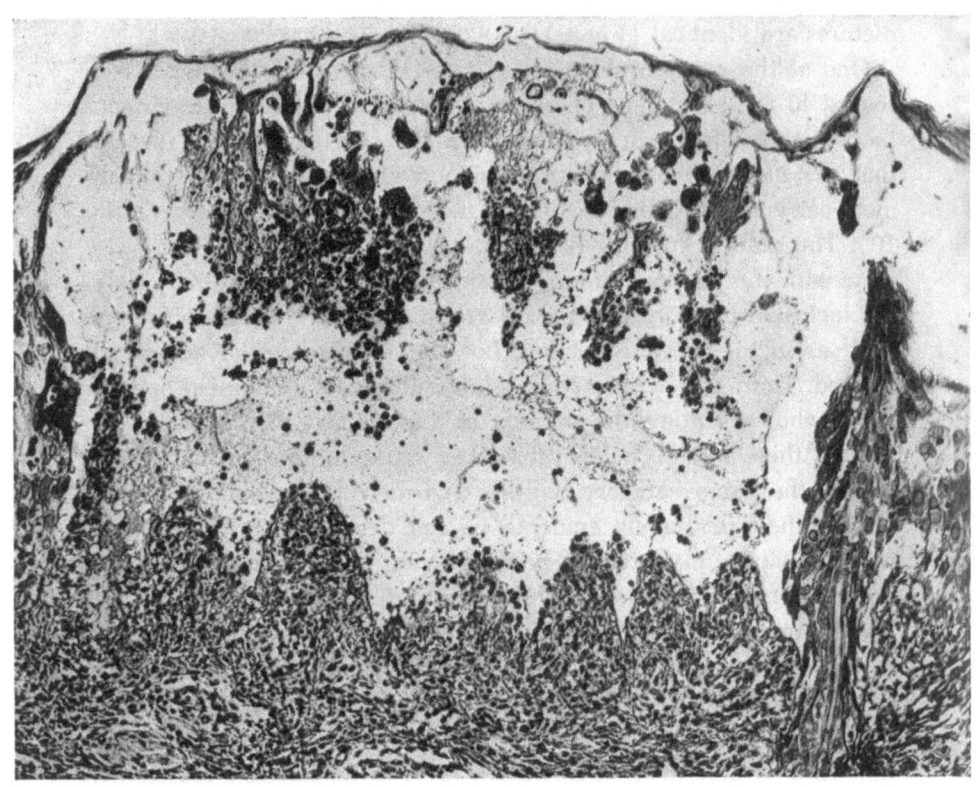

FIGURE 8. HERPES SIMPLEX. BIOPSY OF HUMAN SKIN FROM PATIENT WITH ECZEMA HERPETICUM

Note ballooning degeneration of cells at margins of the lesion, shed epithelial and "virus giant cells" in vesicle fluid, and, in addition, inflammatory cells. Note also that the floor of the vesicle is formed by naked papillae of the corium; there is evidence of infiltration with inflammatory cells but no necrosis of the corium. (Contrast variola, Fig. 4.) Hematoxylin and eosin. Magnification = × 160.

studied herpetic infections of the nervous system and ovulating ovary of the rabbit at twenty-four hours after inoculation, and described a

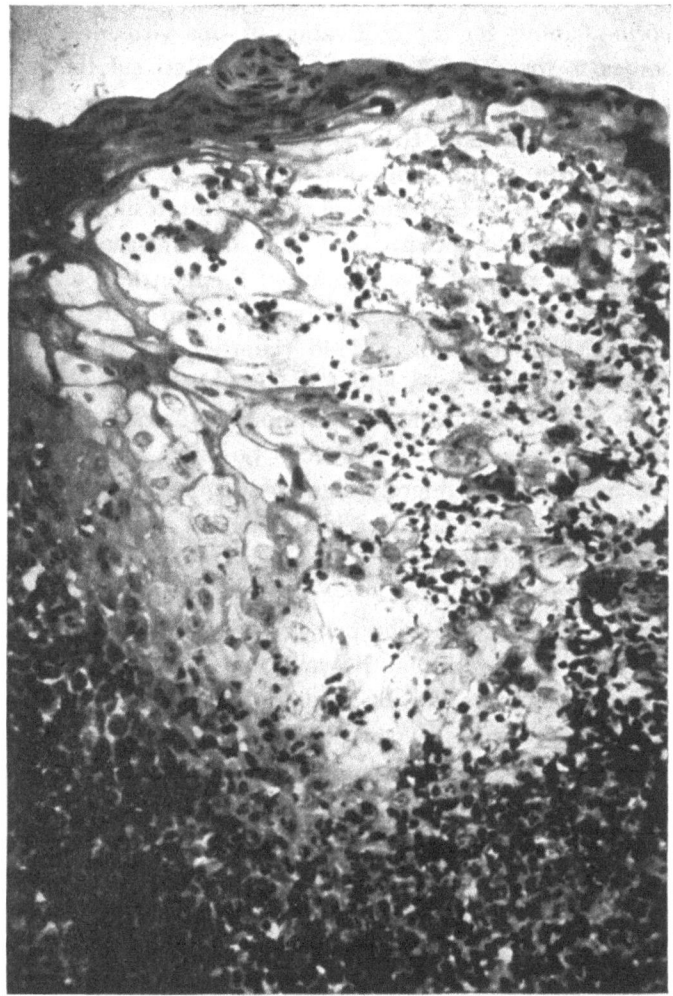

FIGURE 9. HERPES SIMPLEX. BIOPSY OF LESION IN THE MOUTH OF PATIENT SUFFERING FROM ACUTE HERPETIC GINGIVOSTOMATITIS
Note general similarity to lesion of skin except that the vesicle contains less fluid because of leakage due to maceration of the mucous membranes. Hematoxylin and eosin. Magnification = × 160.

cycle of events as follows: Early there appear in the nucleus, several irregular particles staining red with eosin. Later, these coalesce and enlarge to fill the nucleus. At this time they take on a faintly basic stain and appear to be composed of minute bodies of uniform size, packed together.-Again in 1933 Dawson (20), one of the first to use the chorio-allantois for the cultivation of this virus, identified inclusion bodies in the ectodermal cells and pointed out that the largest inclusions stain with basic dyes and appear to be composed of minute basophilic granules. Both these descriptions are compatible with the presence of virus in the inclusions. However, in 1930, Cowdry (21), studying the herpetic infection of the rabbit testicle at forty-eight hours after infection, pointed out that the inclusions were chiefly acidophilic and did not give a positive Feulgen test, although some of the larger ones did give a faintly pink stain with this technique. Lépine and Sautter (22) in 1946 reported that the inclusions of herpes failed to react with either the Feulgen or the toluidine blue stain, this failure indicating the complete absence of nucleic acid. These last two pieces of evidence can be taken to support the view that the inclusions are merely signs of degenerative changes in the nucleus. No time interval after infection was mentioned in Lépine's paper, but the tissue was examined when the classical eosinophilic inclusions were present.

I know of no study with herpes virus comparable to that of Bland and Robinow with vaccinia. However, we have gathered some evidence along this same line by studying the histology of the herpes-infected chorio-allantois at stated intervals after inoculation. No inclusions have been seen before ten hours. From ten to sixteen hours they are scanty, but they increase rapidly thereafter until between twenty and twenty-four hours also every cell contains an intranuclear inclusion. A large number of these are basophilic with hematoxylin and eosin stain, and strongly positive with Feulgen stain. Between forty and forty-eight hours, considerable sloughing has occurred and fewer inclusions are seen. These may vary according to the portion of the lesion examined, so that both basophilic and the classical eosinophilic bodies which are Feulgen- and toluidine-blue negative can be observed. It seems important to bring these findings to your attention as a contrast to Lépine's findings just quoted, since they again emphasize the importance of considering the time element in drawing conclusions as to the presence or absence of virus. It is interesting to note that Baumgartner's successful passages were made

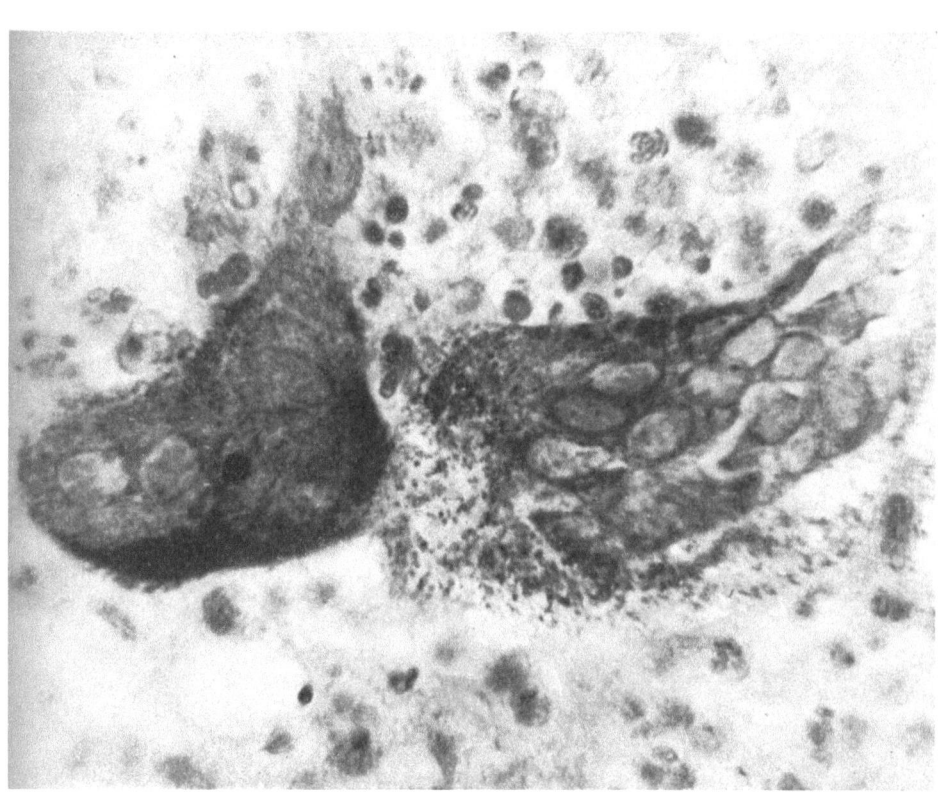

FIGURE 10. HERPES SIMPLEX. RECURRENT LESION IN A NEGRO SHOWING TWO "VIRUS GIANT CELLS" IN WHICH ALL OF THE NUCLEI SHOW THE BASOPHILIC TYPE OF INTRANUCLEAR INCLUSION

Note that the involved cells are the pigment-carrying cells of the basal layer. Hematoxylin and eosin. Magnification = × 900.

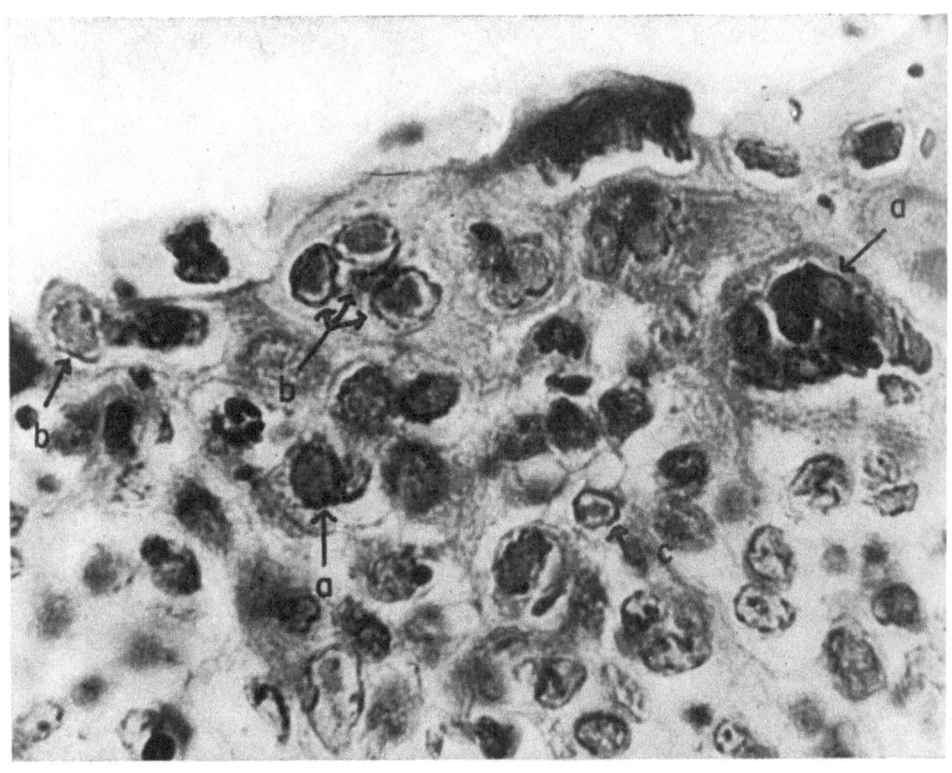

FIGURE 11. HERPES SIMPLEX. RABBIT'S NICTITATING MEMBRANE SHOWING MANY INTRANUCLEAR INCLUSION BODIES: (A) HOMOGENEOUS BASOPHILIC INCLUSION FILLING THE ENLARGED NUCLEUS; (B) INCLUSION BEGINNING TO SHRINK FROM NUCLEAR MEMBRANE AND BECOMING EOSINOPHILIC; (C) CLASSICAL SHRUNKEN EOSINOPHILIC INCLUSION

Hematoxylin and eosin. Magnification = × 900.

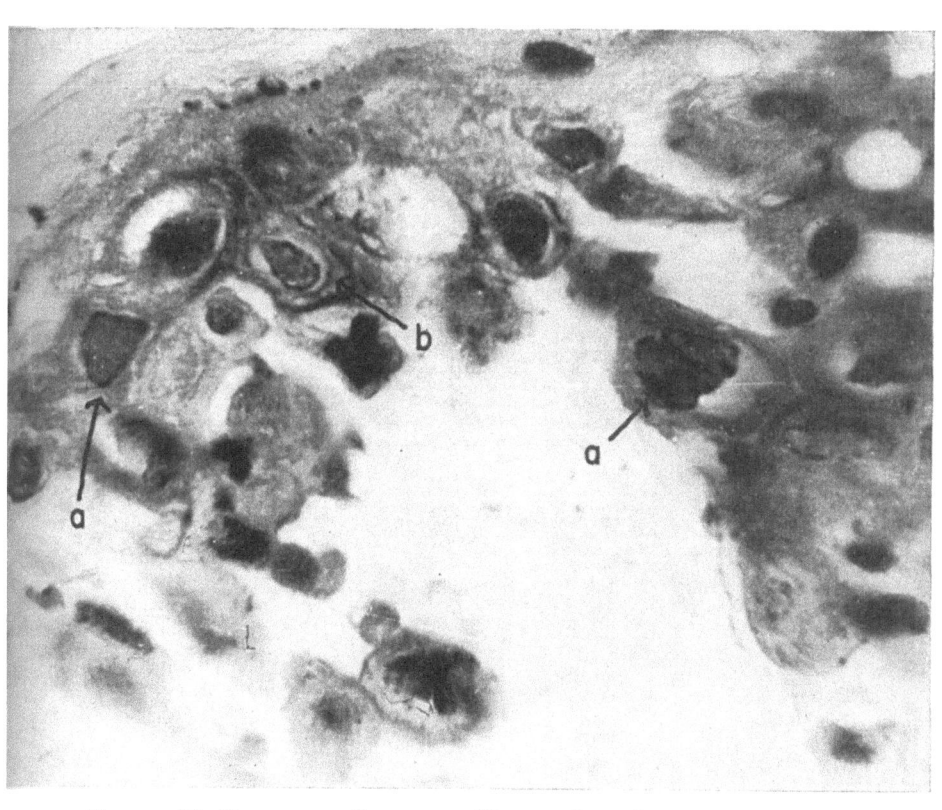

FIGURE 12. VARICELLA. BIOPSY OF HUMAN SKIN SHOWING ROOF OF VESICLE CONTAINING CELLS OF THE MALPIGHIAN LAYER
Cells contain intranuclear inclusion bodies of (a) homogeneous basophilic type; (b) type showing early shrinkage and eosinophilia. Hematoxylin and eosin. Magnification = × 900.

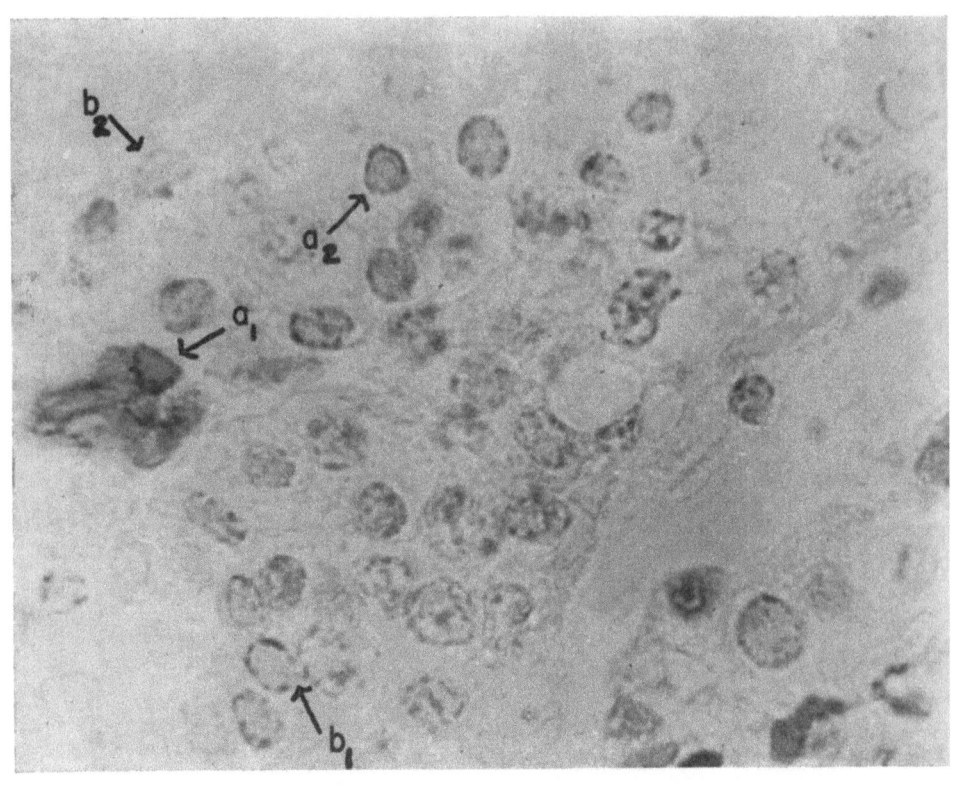

FIGURE 13. HERPES SIMPLEX. CHORIO-ALLANTOIS OF A 12-DAY-OLD EMBRYONATED HEN'S EGG TWENTY-ONE HOURS AFTER INFECTION, SHOWING INTRANUCLEAR INCLUSION BODIES (A_1) STRONGLY FEULGEN-POSITIVE; (A_2) MODERATELY FEULGEN-POSITIVE; (B_1) BARELY FEULGEN-POSITIVE; (B_2) FEULGEN-NEGATIVE
Feulgen. Magnification = × 900.

at a time when, from our histologic findings, the inclusions should have contained a large amount of desoxyribose nucleic acid and, therefore, were not incompatible with the presence of virus.

Some of these points are illustrated in Figs. 11 to 13.

In this discussion of the pathology and pathogenesis of the cutaneous lesions of a selected group of viral diseases, emphasis has been directed toward a consideration of the dynamics of infection in the histological study of viral lesions and the usefulness of the histochemical approach.

REFERENCES

1. Cowdry, E. V., *Laboratory Technique in Biology and Medicine* (2d ed., Baltimore, 1948).
2. Becker, S. W., and M. E. Obermeyer, *Modern Dermatology and Syphilology* (2d ed., Philadelphia, 1947).
3. Torres, C. M., Further studies on the pathology of alastrim and their significance in the variola-alastrim problem, *Proc. Roy. Soc. Med.*, 1935–36, 29:1525.
4. Downie, A. W., and K. R. Dumbell, The isolation and cultivation of variola virus on the chorioallantois of the chick embryo, *J. Path. & Bact.*, 1947, 59:189.
5. Torres, C. M., and J. de Castro Teixeira, A comparison of the inclusion bodies of alastrim and variola vera, *Memorias do Instituto Oswaldo Cruz*, 1935, 30:215.
6. Buist, J. B., The life history of the microorganisms associated with variola and vaccinia, *Proc. Roy. Soc. Edinburgh*, 1886, 13:603.
7. Paschen, E., Was wissen wir über den Vakzinerreger, *Münsch. Med. Wchnschr.*, 1906, 53:2391.
8. van Rooyen, C. E., and A. J. Rhodes, *Virus Diseases of Man*, p. 342 (New York, 1948).
9. Bland, J. O. W., and C. F. Robinow, The inclusion bodies of vaccinia and their relationship to the elementary bodies studied in cultures of the rabbit's cornea, *J. Path. & Bact.*, 1939, 48:381.
10. Hoagland, C. L., G. I. Lavin, J. E. Smadel, and T. M. Rivers, Constituents of elementary bodies of vaccinia, II: Properties of nucleic acid obtained from vaccinia virus, *J. Exp. Med.*, 1940, 72:139.
11. Guarnieri, G., Recherches sur la pathologie et l'étiologie de l'infection vaccinique et varioleuse, *Arch. Ital. de Biol.*, 1893, 19:195.
12. Rake, G., H. Blank, L. L. Coriell, F. P. O. Nagler, and T. F. McNair Scott, The relationship of varicella and herpes zoster, electron microscope studies, *J. Bact.*, 1948, 56:293.
13. Goodpasture, E. W., and K. Anderson, Infection of human skin grafted

on the chorioallantois of chick embryos with the virus of herpes zoster, *Am. J. Path.*, 1944, 20:447.
14. Blank, H., L. L. Coriell, and T. F. McNair Scott, Human skin grafted onto the chorioallantois of the chick embryo for virus cultivation, *Proc. Soc. Exp. Biol. & Med.*, 1948, 69:341.
15. Kundratitz, K., Experimentelle Übertragungen von Herpes Zoster auf Menschen und die Beziehungen von Herpes Zoster zu Varizellen, *Ztschr. f. Kinderheilk.*, 1925, 39:379.
16. Lipschütz, B., Die Einschlusskrankheiten der Haut, Herpes Febrilis. *Handbuch der Haut und Geschlectskrankheiten*, Vol. 2, p. 132 (Berlin, 1932).
17. *Viral and Rickettsial Diseases of Man*, p. 5 (Philadelphia, 1948).
18. Baumgartner, G., Infectionsversuche mit isolierten oxychromatischen Einschlüssen des Herpes, *Schweiz. Med. Wchnschr.*, 1935, 16:759.
19. Goodpasture, E. W., Intranuclear inclusions in experimental herpetic lesions of rabbits, *Am. J. Path.*, 1925, 1:1.
20. Dawson, J. R., Herpetic infection of the chorioallantoic membrane of the chick embryo, *Am. J. Path.*, 1933, 9:1.
21. Cowdry, E. V., A comparison of the intranuclear inclusions produced by herpetic virus and by virus III in rabbits, *Arch. Path.*, 1930, 10:23.
22. Lépine, P., and V. Sautter, Étude histochimique des lesions dues aux ultravirus les acides nucleiques, *Ann. Inst. Pasteur*, 1946, 72:174.

Chapter 8

PATHOGENESIS OF THE VIRAL EXANTHEMS AS EXEMPLIFIED BY MOUSE POX (INFECTIOUS ECTROMELIA OF MICE)

By Frank Fenner, *Walter and Eliza Hall Institute, Melbourne, Australia, and The Rockefeller Institute for Medical Research*

Dr. Scott has described in the preceding chapter the cutaneous lesions of smallpox and chickenpox, two of the human viral exanthems, and he has shown that in each the causative virus can be demonstrated in the skin lesions. When we seek to understand what happens between infection and appearance of the rash several days later, however, we find that very little is known of the pathogenesis of the viral exanthems. This ignorance is due to the fact that the viruses which cause them have not been sucessfully adapted to convenient laboratory animals. Measles and variola viruses have certainly been passed in monkeys and on the chorio-allantoic membrane, but monkeys are expensive animals and simian smallpox and measles are mild diseases. Measles virus fails to cause characteristic lesions in chick embryos, which cannot therefore be used for quantitative studies; and although variola virus causes characteristic focal lesions on the chorio-allantois, this discovery has not been exploited except for the diagnosis of smallpox.

An alternative to the direct study of the pathogenesis of the human viral exanthems is the use as a model of a natural exanthematous disease of a laboratory animal. Following the discovery by Burnet (1) that the virus of infectious ectromelia of mice is closely related to vaccinia virus, it was found (2) that the disease shares with smallpox and generalized vaccinia the characteristic features of the human viral exanthems—a long incubation period and a rash which appears some days after the onset of symptoms. Evidence for the relationship of ectromelia and vaccinia viruses is summarized in Tables 1 and 2.

The first table shows the cross-relationships which exist between the hemagglutinins of vaccinia, variola, and ectromelia viruses. It is apparent that the serum from animals which had recovered from infection with one virus inhibited hemagglutination by the heterologous as well

TABLE 1

HEMAGGLUTININ INHIBITION BY CONVALESCENT SERA

Species	Immunized against	INHIBITION TITER[a] AGAINST	
		Vaccinia HA	Ectromelia HA
Man	Vaccinia	80	40
	Variola	80	80
Rabbit	Vaccinia	160	40
	Ectromelia	40	80
Mouse	Vaccinia	320	160
	Ectromelia	160	640

[a] Titer expressed as reciprocal of highest serum dilution at which four hemagglutinating doses of virus were inhibited.

as the homologous virus, although usually to a lesser extent. Since variola virus was unavailable in Australia, inhibition of variola hemagglutinin by the various sera could not be tested, but serum from a non-vaccinated smallpox patient inhibited vaccinia and ectromelia hemagglutinins to the same degree.

TABLE 2

CROSS-PROTECTION IN ANIMALS IMMUNIZED WITH LIVING VIRUS A FORTNIGHT BEFORE CHALLENGE INOCULATIONS

Species	Immunized with	Challenged with	10^{-1}	10^{-2}	10^{-3}	10^{-4}
Rabbit	Ectromelia 1-V	Vaccinia 1-D	[a]—	—	—	—
	Control	Vaccinia 1-D	+++	+++	++	+
Mouse	Vaccinia 1-N	Ectromelia 1-P	S[b] S	S	S	S
	Controls	Ectromelia 1-P	[b]5 5	5	5	6

[a] — to +++ indicates extent of dermal reaction.
[b] S = survivor at 28 days; figures indicate day of death.

Table 2 shows that the cross-inhibition of hemagglutinins is paralleled by cross-immunity in infected animals. The intravenous inoculation of a large dose of ectromelia virus into rabbits protects them against dermal challenge with vaccinia virus a fortnight later, and inoculation of mice with vaccinia virus protects them against the intraperitoneal inoculation of a dose of ectromelia virus which kills all the control animals.

These facts, plus the resemblances of ectromelia and vaccinia viruses in size and shape and in resistance to heat and drying, make it apparent that infectious ectromelia is indeed mouse pox, the murine representative of the mammalian pox viruses. There is also a close resemblance between the clinical features of mouse pox and those of smallpox. The portal of entry is different, for in smallpox the virus usually enters through the nasopharynx, while in mouse pox the portal of entry consists of small abrasions of the skin. A primary lesion develops at the site of entry of the virus, and as this is the first evidence of infection, it indicates the end of the incubation period.

Within two or three days of the appearance of the primary lesion the infected mouse usually dies, with extensive necrosis of the liver and spleen, or it develops a generalized rash. The earliest lesions of the rash are small papules, and sections show that the majority of the epidermal cells in such papules contain inclusion bodies. After a day or so the papules ulcerate, and sections then show that the epidermal cells have become necrotic, forming adherent scabs, and the corium is now edematous and invaded by numerous lymphocytes.

About seven days elapse between exposure to infection or the inoculation of a small dose of virus into the foot pad, and the appearance of the primary lesions, so that the incubation period in the natural disease and its experimental counterpart is about a week (Table 3).

TABLE 3

LENGTH OF INCUBATION PERIOD IN MOUSE POX

	Number of Mice	Length of Incubation Period (to Appearance of Primary Lesion)
24-hour exposure	32	6.8 ± 1.7 days
Pad inoculation (500 ID_{50})	23	7.2 ± 1.2 days

Summing up, therefore: Mouse pox is a valid model of the human viral exanthems, for it is caused by a virus closely related to one of them, it has a relatively long incubation period, and a few days after the onset of symptoms a rash appears. Evidence of local virus multiplication is present in the lesions of the rash.

To study the pathogenesis of mouse pox, advantage was taken of the fact that the virus can be titrated on the chorio-allantois of the chick embryo, as well as in mice. Groups of mice were infected either by rubbing virus into the skin or by inoculating small doses into the foot pad. At intervals of hours or days they were killed and the virus content of various organs titrated (3).

TABLE 4

SPREAD OF ECTROMELIA VIRUS THROUGH THE MOUSE AFTER VIRUS IS RUBBED ONTO ONE EAR

Material	Hours after Infection		Days after Infection			
	4	8	1	2	3	5
Ear	+	+	++	+++	+++	++++
Regional: Lymph node	0	+	+	++	+++	++++
Blood	0	0	0	0	+	++
Liver	....	....	0	0	++	++++
Spleen	....	....	0	0	++	++++

As the data recorded in Table 4 indicate, the first site, other than the portal of entry, from which virus was isolated was the regional lymph node, and three days after the mice have been infected virus was also found in the liver, spleen, and blood. Daily titration of the virus content of the inoculated foot, the spleen, the blood, and the skin of mice infected by the inoculation of a smaller dose of virus in the foot pad gave results which are recorded graphically in Fig. 1. The organs of two mice were titrated separately each day, and essentially similar curves were obtained in two other similar experiments.

It is apparent that infection spread through the mouse in a definite order: local lesion, regional lymph node, spleen and liver, blood stream, and skin. In each tissue and organ the virus concentration increased logarithmically for a few days, reached a stationary phase, and then fell. Macroscopic lesions of the foot, spleen, and skin were detected only when the virus titer in each had almost reached its maximum.

These observations may be interpreted as shown diagrammatically in Fig. 2. Infection with ectromelia virus occurs by the introduction of a few virus particles into the skin of the mouse, either naturally through an abrasion or by inoculation. Within eight hours of the establishment of infection, virus passes to the regional lymph node, within which it multiplies for a few days. Necrosis of cells in the lymph node then liberates virus, which enters the blood stream but is immediately taken up by the phagocytes of the liver and spleen and possibly the bone marrow. Contiguous cells of these organs are infected, with a great increase in the concentration of virus. Virus is then liberated

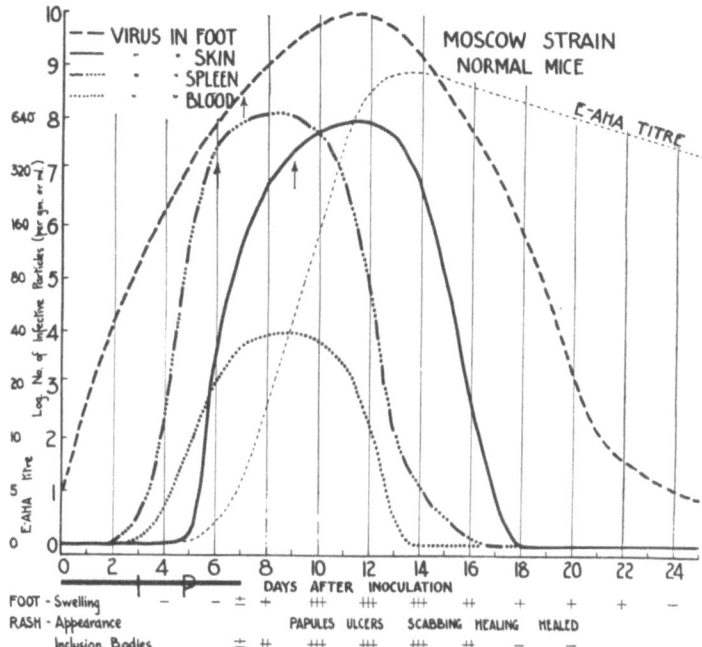

FIGURE 1. GROWTH CURVES OF ECTROMELIA VIRUS IN VARIOUS TISSUES AND ORGANS AFTER THE INOCULATION OF A SMALL DOSE INTO THE FOOT PAD

Arrows indicate time at which macroscopic signs of infection were first observed.

directly into the blood stream by necrosis of the infected cells which line the sinusoids of those organs. This secondary viremia, which is first evident on the fourth day after infection, results in widespread focal infection of the epidermal cells, virus being first detected in the skin on the sixth day. By this time the titer of virus in the primary lesion has reached a high level, for the first time there is obvious edema at the site of entry of the virus, and the incubation period has come to an end.

The edema increases and ulceration occurs, and the mouse then liberates virus into the environment; i. e., it is infective. Meanwhile virus multiplication in the liver and spleen is rapid, and may be so destructive of the cells of these organs that both become almost completely necrotic and the mouse dies. Virus multiplication in the skin

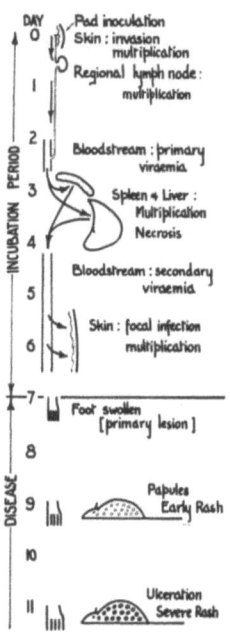

FIGURE 2. DIAGRAMMATIC REPRESENTATION OF THE PATHOGENESIS OF MOUSE POX

lags behind that in the liver and spleen, for the skin is not infected until the period of the secondary viremia occurring from the fourth day onward. If death occurs before the eighth or ninth day, as deaths in the acute stage usually do, no skin lesions are found, but the virus content of the skin is high and microscopic sections may show many inclusions bodies within the epidermal cells, the distribution of groups of infected cells being focal. If multiplication of virus in the liver and spleen is less extreme and the animals survive the acute phase of the disease, edema of the epidermal cells becomes clinically obvious as pale macules, and these rapidly become papular and ulcerate because of necrosis of the superficial cells. The massive liberation of virus which then occurs is responsible for the high infectivity of the disease at this stage. By this time the circulating antibody has reached a high titer and skin sensitization to the virus can also be elicited. Antibody probably prevents the virus from infecting new cells, the virus content of all organs and tissues rapidly falls, and the infected animal recovers.

If we now consider briefly what is known of the pathogenesis of the human viral exanthems (4), we see that the facts accord with the hypothesis just outlined. The analogy is closest in generalized vaccinia or inoculation variola or chickenpox, for the portal of entry is the skin, the incubation period (to the onset of symptoms) varies from four to eight days, and the rash appears between two and four days later. It seems altogether likely that between infection and the widespread focal multiplication of the virus in the skin which causes the rash, there must be a period of multiplication in some internal organ so that prolonged viremia can occur. The most likely foci for multiplication are those organs in which virus entering the blood in small amounts is readily taken up by macrophages, and after multiplication is readily released again into the blood stream; i. e., the speen, liver, or bone marrow.

In ordinary smallpox, chickenpox, measles, and rubella the portal of entry is probably the nasopharynx, and the longer incubation period of these diseases may be partially accounted for by a delay between implantation of the virus on a mucous surface and its entry into the blood stream, compared with the course of events in direct intradermal inoculation. Probably the reproduction rates of the different viruses are also different. But here again the long symptomless incubation period and the appearance of a rash which indicates blood-stream dissemination of large amounts of virus can best be accounted for by some such scheme as is shown in Fig. 2.

Such a hypothesis also provides an explanation for the durable immunity of the viral exanthems, for the long period of secondary viremia insures massive and universal distribution of virus to all the antibody-forming organs, and the necessity of the passage of virus through the lymph and blood stream before infection of an internal focus can occur allows circulating antibody to exert its effect during any second infection.

In some textbooks of medicine the description of the symptoms of smallpox and measles is divided into periods of incubation, invasion, and eruption. If the pathogenesis of those diseases is as we suggest here, this description is obviously incorrect. "Invasion" presumably means either the entry of virus into the blood stream, or the invasion of organs by virus spread through the blood stream. Both these events occur during the incubation period and do not cause symptoms.

SUMMARY

There is good reason to believe that mouse pox is a valid model for the study of the pathogenesis of the acute exanthems. Quantitative studies of the virus titer of different organs and tissues of infected mice showed that in mouse pox there was a regular stepwise progress of virus from the portal of entry, through the regional lymph nodes to the blood stream, whence it was removed, presumably by the macrophages of the liver and spleen. Multiplication in these organs occurred and virus was released again into the blood stream in large amounts. Focal infection of the skin and occasionally of other organs followed and after a further period of multiplication the virus concentration of the skin reached a high level and lesions of the skin appeared.

It is suggested that the pathogenesis of the human viral exanthems follows a similar basic pattern.

REFERENCES

1. Burnet, F. M., and W. E. Boake, The relationship between the virus of infectious ectromelia of mice and vaccinia virus, *J. Immunol.*, 1946, 53:1.
2. Fenner, Frank, The epizootic behavior of mousepox (infectious ectromelia), *Brit. J. Exp. Path.*, 1948, 29:69.
3. Fenner, Frank, The clinical features of mousepox (infectious ectromelia of mice) and the pathogenesis of the disease, *J. Path. Bact.*, 1949.
4. Fenner, Frank, The pathogenesis of the acute exanthems: An interpretation based upon experimental investigations with mousepox (infectious ectromelia of mice), *Lancet*, 1948, 2:915.

Chapter 9

CARDIAC LESIONS PRODUCED BY VIRUSES[1]

By John M. Pearce, *Department of Pathology, Long Island College of Medicine, Hoagland Laboratory, and Departments of Pathology and Surgery, Cornell University Medical College, New York Hospital–Cornell Medical Center*

During the past several years it has been possible to show that a filtrable virus when introduced into the animal body by a peripheral route can specifically infect the heart and there produce anatomical lesions and functional derangement, that this ability is not the property of a single virus but is common to several, and finally that an important factor in inducing the cardiac localization of virus is a decrease in the amount of oxygen supplied to the heart. This portion of the symposium is an attempt to describe the experiments and their results by which these conclusions have been reached and to demonstrate the variety of cardiac lesions obtained.

The initial observations were made with virus III in several rabbits that had had their hearts punctured by a hollow needle in the process of obtaining sterile blood for use in tissue cultures. A few minutes after withdrawal of the needle a saline suspension of virus III infected tissue had been injected into each testis. This double procedure was done with no intention of producing cardiac lesions but solely as an economy measure by which the same animal could be used both as a source of normal serum and for routine virus passage. The animals were killed four to five days later to obtain the testicular passage virus. Routine autopsies were performed, and when the hearts were examined microscopically they were found to contain widespread inflammatory lesions characterized by the intranuclear inclusion bodies typical of virus III infection. Although there has never been any difficulty in recovering virus from the hearts, this inclusion body has been most useful in the studies to be described, since it identifies the bacteriologically

[1] The work summarized here was aided by grants from the United Hospital Fund of New York and the Life Insurance Medical Research Fund.

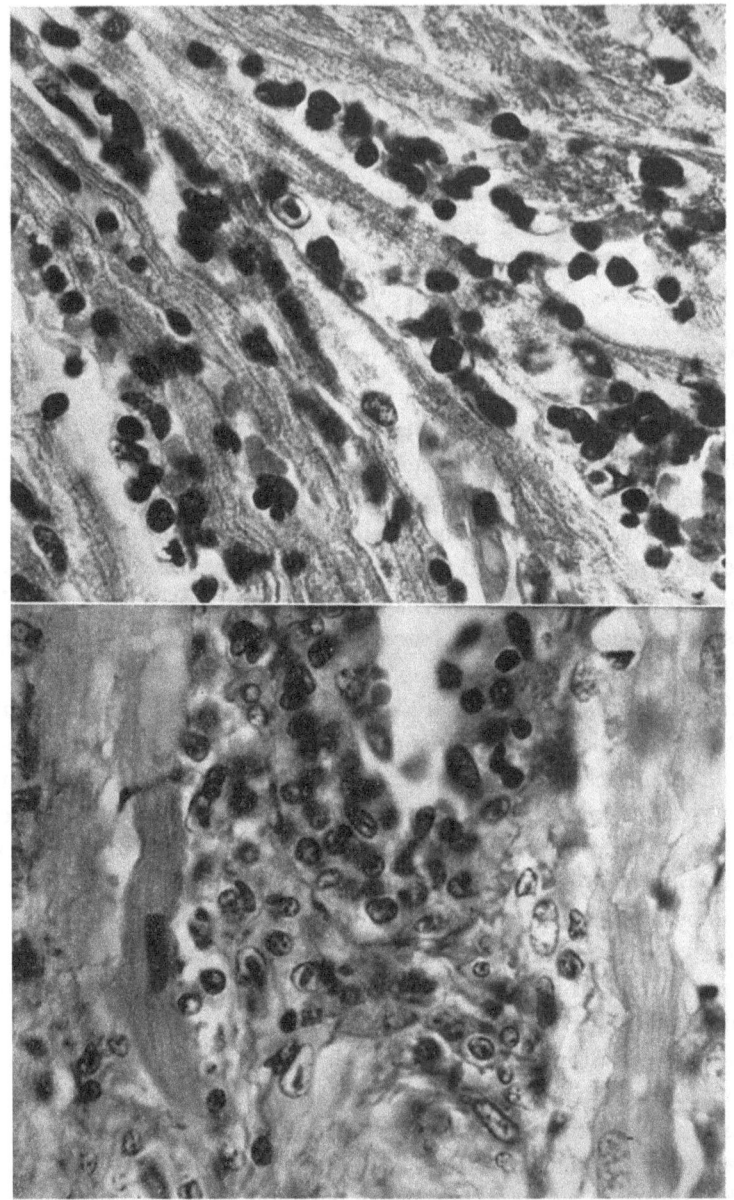

FIGURE 1. INTRANUCLEAR INCLUSION BODIES OF VIRUS III IN AREAS OF LEUCOCYTIC INFILTRATION AND FIBROBLASTIC PROLIFERATION IN THE MYOCARDIUM
Hematoxylin and eosin. Magnification = × 700.

sterile lesion as being viral in origin and does away with the necessity for the more laborious procedure of demonstrating virus by further animal inoculation in every instance. As can be seen in Fig. 1, it is a definite and striking structure, consisting of a darkly acidophilic mass that lies in the center of a swollen nucleus surrounded by a pale or vacuolated area, at the periphery of which the scant remaining chromatin is situated just inside the prominent nuclear membrane. The effect is that of a halo. The inclusion tends to conform to the shape of the nucleus, being round in round nuclei and elongated or oval in oval nuclei.

The finding of the cardiac lesions in the rabbits that had been bled led to the examination of the hearts of those animals that had had no treatment other than the intratesticular inoculation of virus III. In a rare heart a focus of mild cellular infiltration with a few inclusions could be found, but these lesions were never impressive and were usually inconsequential. It was quite obvious that the occurrence of serious inflammatory lesions occurred almost exclusively in those rabbits that had had their hearts punctured just prior to viral inoculation.

Plunging a needle through the ventricular wall is an extremely drastic and unphysiological method of producing cardiac localization of virus, even though in the uninfected animal the passage of the needle alone seldom leaves any residual damage demonstrable after a four-day interval. Since myocarditis or endocarditis of viral origin would be much more significant if the procedure used to induce the cardiac localization of the infecting agent more closely approached conditions that might occur spontaneously in the life of the animal, a search was begun for such a method. Two procedures were found almost at once: the intravenous administration of betahypophamine ("pitressin") and the intravenous injection of solutions of gum acacia, both of which, but especially the latter, were followed by a high incidence of a carditis characterized by its severity. A report by Nedzel (1), in which he showed that pitressin given intravenously brought about localization of bacteria on the heart valves of dogs, with bacterial endocarditis resulting, led to the use of this drug in the hope that a similar phenomenon would bring about a virus-induced vegetation. The use of acacia was suggested by the work of Clark and Svec (2), in which they were able to produce bacterial endocarditis by

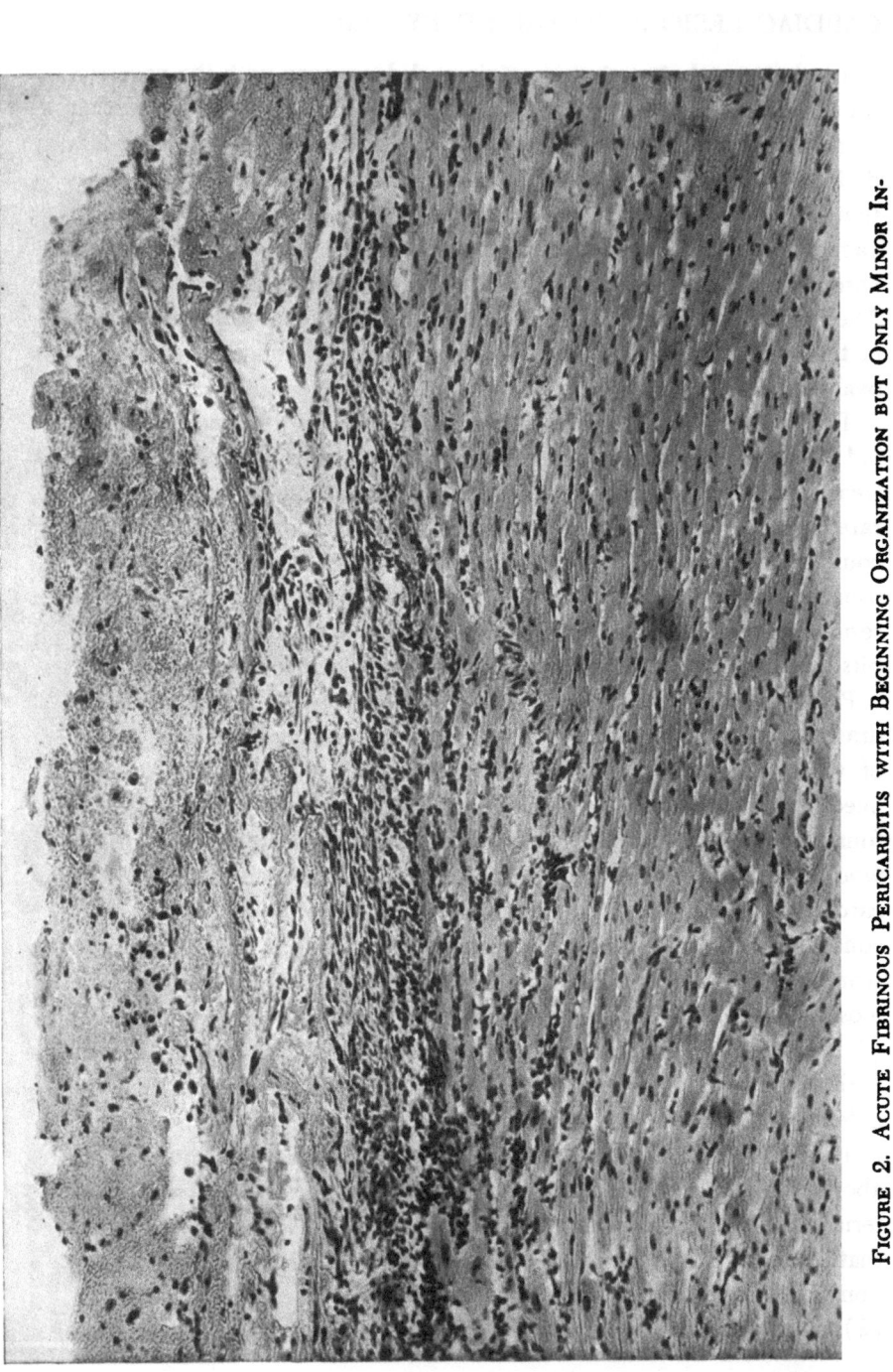

FIGURE 2. ACUTE FIBRINOUS PERICARDITIS WITH BEGINNING ORGANIZATION BUT ONLY MINOR INFLAMMATION OF THE UNDERLYING MYOCARDIUM. FIVE DAYS AFTER INTRAVENOUS INJECTION OF VIRUS III. Hematoxylin and eosin. Magnification = × 150.

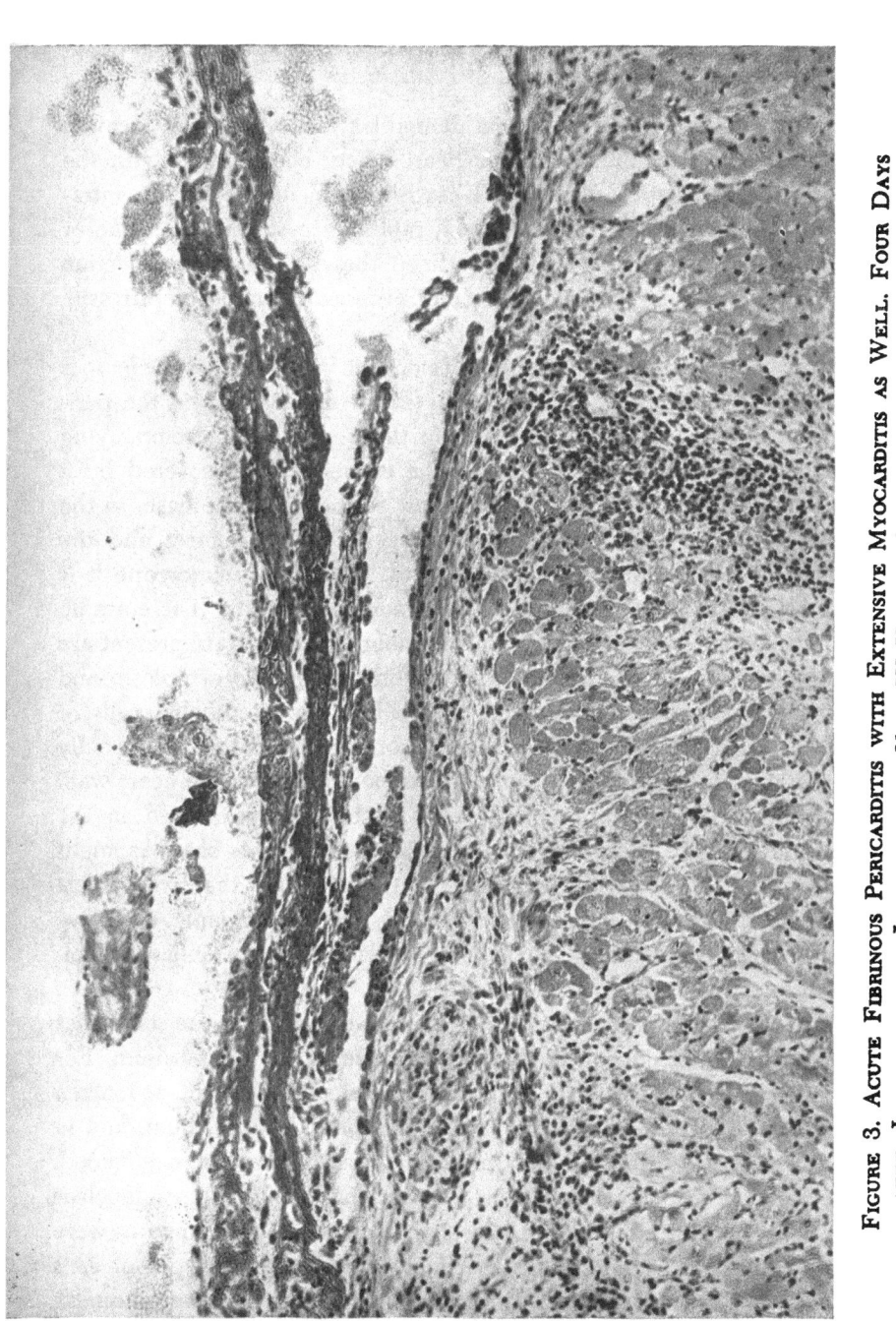

FIGURE 3. ACUTE FIBRINOUS PERICARDITIS WITH EXTENSIVE MYOCARDITIS AS WELL. FOUR DAYS AFTER INTRATESTICULAR INOCULATION OF VIRUS III. Hematoxylin and eosin. Magnification = × 150.

preceding the infecting dose of bacteria by a large intravenous injection of gum acacia.

The accompanying illustrations demonstrate the type and location of the lesions encountered in the heart when, concomitant with the peripheral inoculation of virus III (intravenous, intratesticular, intranasal, subcutaneous, or intradermal), rabbits are subjected to one or the other of the three procedures outlined above—intravenous injection of hypertonic gum acacia solution, intravenous injection of pitressin, or cardiac puncture.

Pericarditis is the least common lesion but when it does occur it is quite striking (Figs. 2, 3). The exudate and the reaction in the pericardium closely resemble that seen in the pericarditis accompanying rheumatic fever in human beings. The entire heart is covered by a coating of dull, sticky fibrin that is most abundant at the base, in the crevices around the auricles, and between these structures and the ventricles in the interventricular grooves. Under the microscope it is apparent that this is an almost pure fibrinous pericarditis. There are no polymorphonuclear leucocytes, and the leucocytes that are present are chiefly mononuclear cells that have slightly basophilic cytoplasm and frequently suggest desquamated or proliferating mesothelial cells of the epicardium. Almost always there is some organization, and usually a rich growth of fibroblasts extends into the fibrin from the heart wall. Inclusion bodies can be found both in the cells enmeshed in the fibrinous exudate and in the new connective tissue at its base. As might be expected, pericarditis occurred in those hearts that were most severely affected in other respects, and not uncommonly extensive areas of myocarditis lay immediately adjacent to the inflamed epicardium.

Lesions of the endocardium, both mural and valvular, are somewhat more frequently encountered than are those of the pericardium. For instance, in one early series of experiments thirteen of seventeen affected animals developed lesions of the mural endocardium, and in seven of these thirteen one or more of the valves was also inflamed. The affected valve was thickened by an infiltration of mononuclear cells, by a proliferation of fibroblasts among which mitotic figures were numerous, and by edema. In the nuclei of both these types of cells there were inclusion bodies (Fig. 4). At times the chordae tendineae

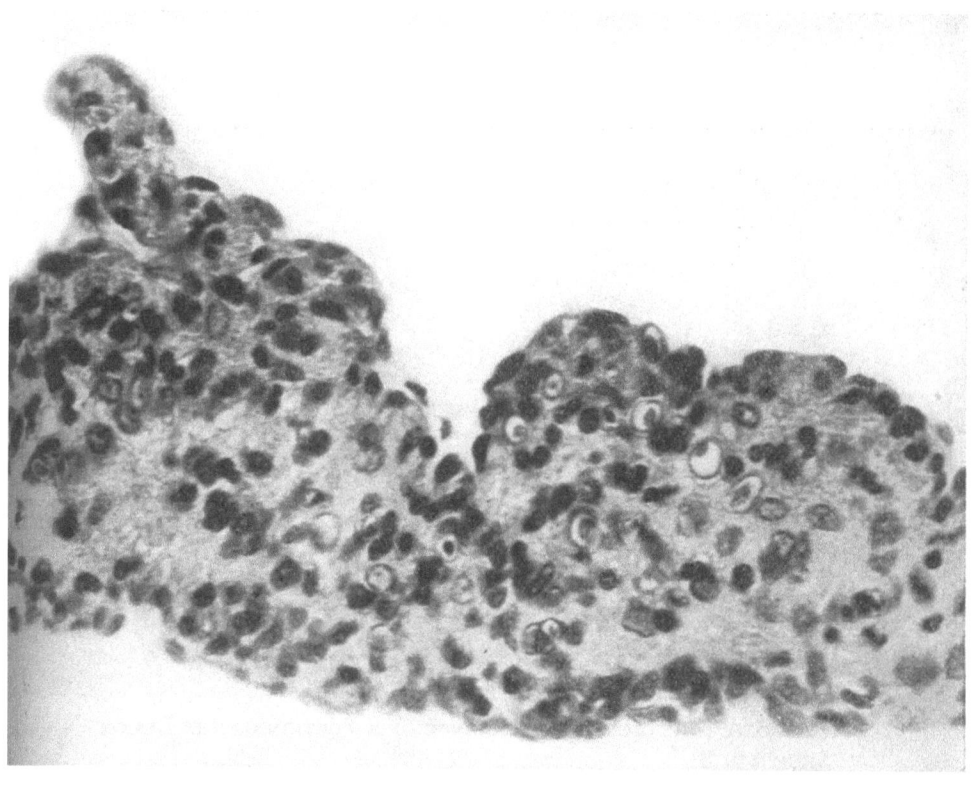

FIGURE 4. VIRUS III INCLUSION BODIES IN NUCLEI OF CELLS IN THICK-
ENED AND INFILTRATED TRICUSPID VALVE

Hematoxylin and eosin. Magnification = × 450. (Figs. 4, 7, 8, 9, and 13 have appeared previously in the *Archives of Pathology* [1939, 28:836; 1942, 34:322, 324, 325; 1947, 44:110]. They are reproduced here by the courtesy of that journal.)

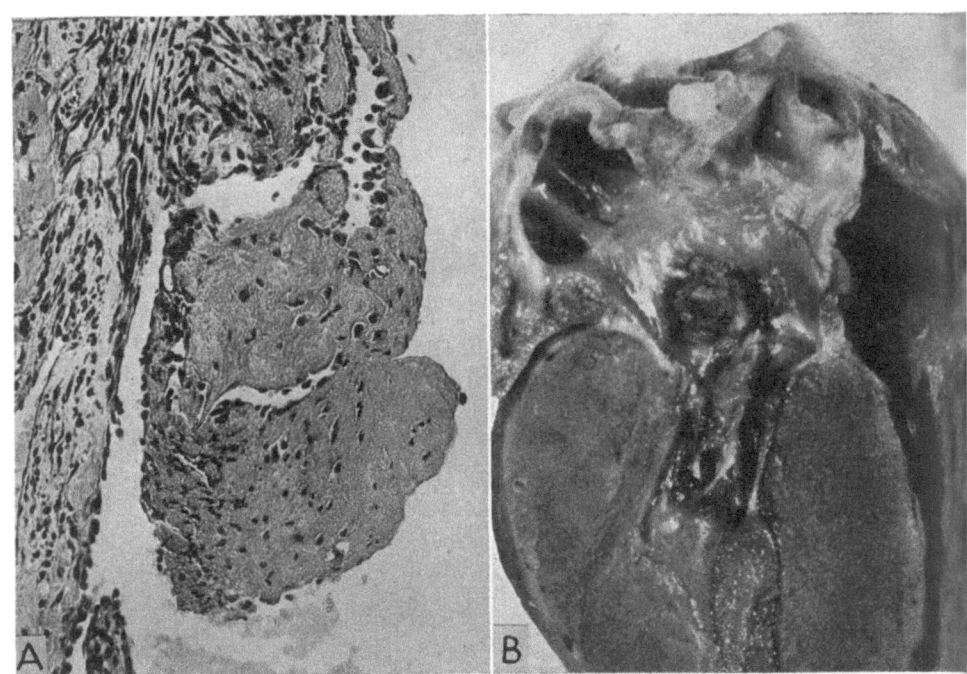

FIGURE 5. A. MICROSCOPIC APPEARANCE OF A PORTION OF THE LESION SHOWN IN B
B. LARGE, LOOSELY ATTACHED NONBACTERIAL FIBRINOID VEGETATIONS ON BASILAR PORTION OF MITRAL VALVE
Magnification = × 3.
A partially organized mass of fibrinoid vegetations containing neither bacteria nor polymorphonuclear leucocytes is loosely attached to the endocardium. Hematoxylin and eosin. Magnification = × 150.

showed diffuse or nodular thickening and infiltration similar to that in the valve proper.

Fibrinoid vegetations were occasionally encountered. Fig. 5 shows a lesion on the mitral valve of a rabbit inoculated intratesticularly with

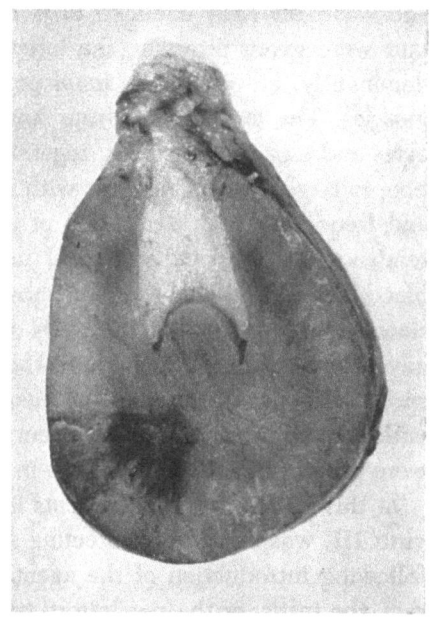

FIGURE 6. INFARCT IN THE KIDNEY OF THE ANIMAL WHOSE HEART IS ILLUSTRATED IN FIG. 5, A AND B. Magnification = × 3.

virus III five days before it was killed and examined. Bacterial cultures of blood taken from the marginal ear vein just before death were negative. Fibroblasts and mononuclear cells at the base of this large vegetation contained intranuclear inclusions. That it was only loosely attached to the valve is indicated not only by its appearance in the picture but by the presence of an infarct in the kidney (Fig. 6) that presumably was caused by an embolic occlusion of a renal artery.

In the animals treated with acacia or pitressin the mural endocarditis was never extensive, consisting solely of plaque-like collections of mononuclear cells and lymphocytes, again with occasional inclusion-bearing nuclei. In those hearts that had been entered by the bleeding needle, mural thrombi with necrosis of the underlying endocardium and intense inflammation of the myocardium were found at points that have been interpreted as the site of puncture of the ventricular wall. It must be emphasized again that no such lesion occurred in animals that have been bled but have not been inoculated with virus.

The muscle is the part of the heart that is most frequently involved and most seriously altered. In the rabbits prepared by the injection of acacia into a vein, the myocarditis was distributed equally between auricles and ventricles but was much more severe on the right side and was frequently confined to it. On the other hand, in the animals that were given pitressin, the left ventricular wall was affected predominantly, especially the inner portion of it and the large papillary muscles. The lesions vary from small nodular collections of lymphocytes and mononuclear cells, together with some fibroblastic proliferation, to large areas of necrosis with much new growth of fibrous tissue and frequently with deposition of calcium. (Fig. 10). There is some tendency for the smaller foci of inflammation to be situated beside blood vessels. Swelling and necrosis of perivascular collagen occasionally takes place, but the walls of arteries or arterioles never show any definite change. In many of the pitressin-treated animals a widespread diffuse infiltration of the myocardium without any necrosis and with few nodular aggregates occurred. Intranuclear inclusion bodies were present in a variety of cells in all these lesions (Fig. 1).

At this stage of the experiments it had become obvious that a virus, virus III, was capable of infecting and producing lesions in the heart following introduction of the agent by way of the venous blood, the skin, the testis, or the respiratory tract if the animal was prepared by accompanying the inoculation with some other suitable procedure. From this observation two pressing questions arose.

The first question was whether this ability of virus III to localize in the heart and there cause inflammation is peculiar to it or is common to a variety of viruses. Is it a specific quality peculiar to this particular virus or is it a property shared with a number of dissimilar and unrelated viruses that may act similarly under the same conditions?

The second question concerns the fact that although it is not surprising that such a crude and unphysiologic procedure as cardiac puncture induces circulating virus to lodge in the heart, it is most puzzling that two such physically and pharmacologically dissimilar substances as an extract containing betahypophamine ("pitressin") and a solution of acacia should have a similar effect. What is the action on the heart that these two substances have in common that causes that organ to be more susceptible to infection and damage by virus?

CARDIAC LESIONS CAUSED BY OTHER VIRUSES THAN VIRUS III

Arbitrarily it was decided to approach first the problem of the specificity of virus III. Five other viruses were selected for study on the basis of the ease with which they can infect the rabbit and their possession of characteristic or identifying histological reactions. These five were vaccine virus, two strains of fibroma virus—Shope's original strain A and Andrewes' inflammatory strain—pseudorabies virus, and virus myxomatosum.[1] Since the intravenous injections of acacia solutions had brought about the highest incidence of cardiac involvement by virus III this method of preparation was used in the experiments with these other agents. Thirty-five to 50 c.c. of a 20 percent solution of sterile acacia in 0.85 percent sodium chloride was injected into the marginal ear vein of ten animals in each of five groups of fifteen, and each group of fifteen was then inoculated intratesticularly with one of the five viruses. The results (Table 1) closely parallel those obtained when virus III was used, a high incidence of carditis occurring in infection by all these different viruses. In the case of the myxoma virus the percentage incidence of lesions in this small series is the same in the control group that received no acacia as in the prepared group, but it must be emphasized that in all instances the lesions in the hearts of the controls did not approach the number or magnitude of those in the prepared group.

[1] The myxoma virus, the pseudorabies virus, and the two strains of fibroma virus were procured from Doctor Richard Shope, of the Rockefeller Institute. The myxoma virus was the strain originally obtained from Doctor Arthur Moses, of the Oswaldo Cruz Institute, in Brazil, and used by both H. R. Hobbs (*Am. J. Hyg.*, 1928, 8:800) and T. M. Rivers (*J. Exp. Med.*, 1930, 51:965) and maintained by Doctor Shope in the laboratories of the Rockefeller Institute in Princeton since 1932. The strain A fibroma virus was that originally isolated by R. E. Shope (*J. Exp. Med.*, 1932, 56:793). The inflammatory fibroma virus was the variant described by C. H. Andrewes (*J. Exp. Med.*, 1936, 63:157) and sent by him to Shope. The vaccine virus which was used was a highly virulent strain isolated by me from a spontaneously infected rabbit in 1938 (*J. Infect. Dis.*, 1940, 66:130). The pseudorabies virus was the Hungarian strain which had been sent to Shope by Aujeszky from Budapest in 1930.

The myxoma virus and the strain A fibroma virus had been maintained by both intratesticular and subcutaneous serial passage through rabbits and by storage in 50 percent glycerin. The vaccine virus and the inflammatory fibroma virus had been carried by testicular passage and storage in glycerin, and the pseudorabies virus, by serial intracerebral inoculation and storage in glycerin.

The character of the lesion varied in detail with the peculiarities of the inciting agent, but the general disease picture and the location of lesions were the same in all. Myocarditis predominated in all infections;

TABLE 1

INCIDENCE OF CARDIAC INVOLVEMENT IN RABBITS DURING INFECTION BY SEVERAL VIRUSES

Virus	Infected Rabbits	Number with Significant Lesions of the Heart	Percentage
Rabbits Prepared by Intravenous Injection of a Solution of Acacia			
Vaccine virus	10	8	80
Pseudorabies virus	10	7	70
Fibroma virus (inflammatory strain)	10	8	80
Myxoma virus	10	6	60
Fibroma virus (strain A)	10	7	70
Rabbits Which Had not Received the Solution of Acacia			
Vaccine virus	5	1	20
Pseudorabies virus	5	2	40
Fibroma virus (inflammatory strain)	5	1	20
Myxoma virus	5	3	60
Fibroma virus (strain A)	5	0	0

in vaccinia and pseudorabies the valves also were frequently affected. Vaccine virus tends to produce numerous small nodular lesions in the myocardium consisting of small foci of necrosis infiltrated and surrounded by mononuclear and polymorphonuclear leucocytes (Fig. 7), but in some hearts there was a diffuse infiltration of large areas of myocardium by leucocytes. In the mitral and tricuspid valves there occurred an interstitial infiltration of leucocytes, together with edema and a proliferation of fibroblasts, which often resulted in marked thickening of the flap (Fig. 8). Hemorrhages were commonly found in the substance of the cusps, but in this series fibrinoid vegetations were not encountered on their surfaces.

In the animals infected with the pseudorabies virus the lesion was again predominantly a myocarditis, and except for the presence of the intranuclear inclusion bodies characteristic of this disease (Fig. 9) was not dissimilar to that seen in vaccinia. Somewhat patchy but frequently confluent areas of leucocytic infiltration, disappearance of muscle cells, and fibrosis were spread through the right side of the heart. Rows of

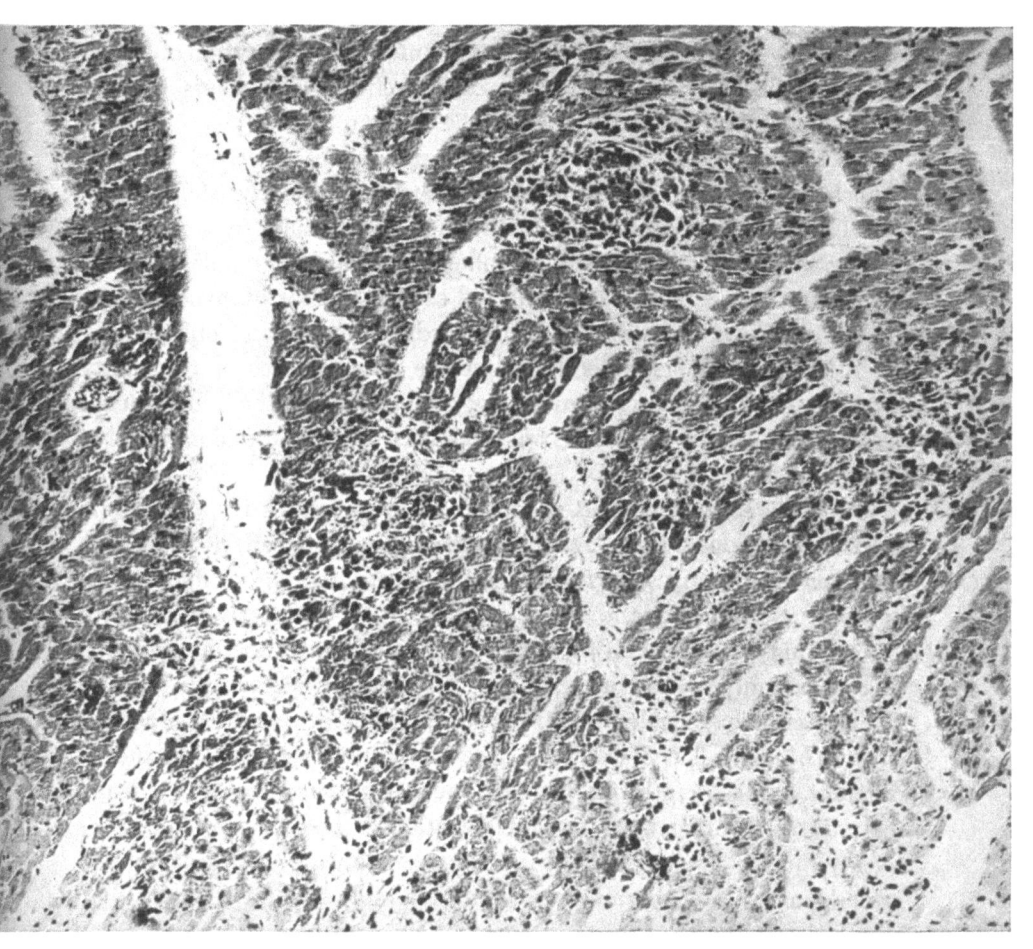

FIGURE 7. VACCINIA MYOCARDITIS. SMALL FOCI OF MUSCLE NECROSIS SURROUNDED BY NODULAR COLLECTIONS OF MONONUCLEAR PHAGOCYTES AND PROLIFERATING FIBROBLASTS
Hematoxylin and eosin. Magnification = × 128. (See note, Fig. 4.)

swollen endothelial cells containing intranuclear inclusion bodies lined parts of the auricles.

Although the inflammatory fibroma virus killed none of the inoculated animals, leucocytic infiltration and necrosis were severe in many hearts and were characteristically accompanied by proliferation of large basophilic fibroblasts. Calcification of necrotic muscle fibers was a common feature (Fig. 10).

The myocarditis of the myxoma group was characterized by the typical myxomatous tissue reaction. Large, irregularly stellate or spindle-shaped basophilic cells with huge, pale nuclei in which the chromatin was finely stippled or collected in larger granules at the prominent nuclear membrane, replaced extensive areas of myocardium (Fig. 11). These cells filled the endocardial crevices and obliterated the columnae carneae, smoothing out the inner surface of the right ventricle. In spite of the destruction of cardiac muscle fibers, the thickness of the wall of the heart was increased by the abundant newly formed tissue.

The strain A fibroma virus produced the least impressive alteration. The valves, endocardium, and pericardium were not affected. In the right ventricular muscle there was a diffuse proliferation of fibroblasts between muscle fibers and larger scar-like areas of fibrosis (Fig. 12).

Including virus III with these five additional viruses there are, then, at least six viruses that are capable of infecting the heart of the rabbit. These six differ considerably from one another in several characteristics. The clinical course of the diseases caused by them are quite different. Virus III infection is mild. There is no objective sign of it in most instances other than a slight elevation of body temperature for twenty-four to seventy-two hours. Recovery always occurs. Pseudorabies runs an even shorter course but invariably ends in death on the third or the fourth day after inoculation, and the temperature is markedly elevated. Myxomatosis also is almost always fatal, but in this disease the animals survive for several weeks and have visible involvement of various mucocutaneous junctions and a blinding purulent ophthalmitis. At autopsy lesions are found in many viscera. Vaccinia in the rabbit is a severe and frequently fatal disease. The two strains of fibroma virus produce diseases that are never fatal but that differ in duration.

The reaction of the host tissues to these six invaders is extremely

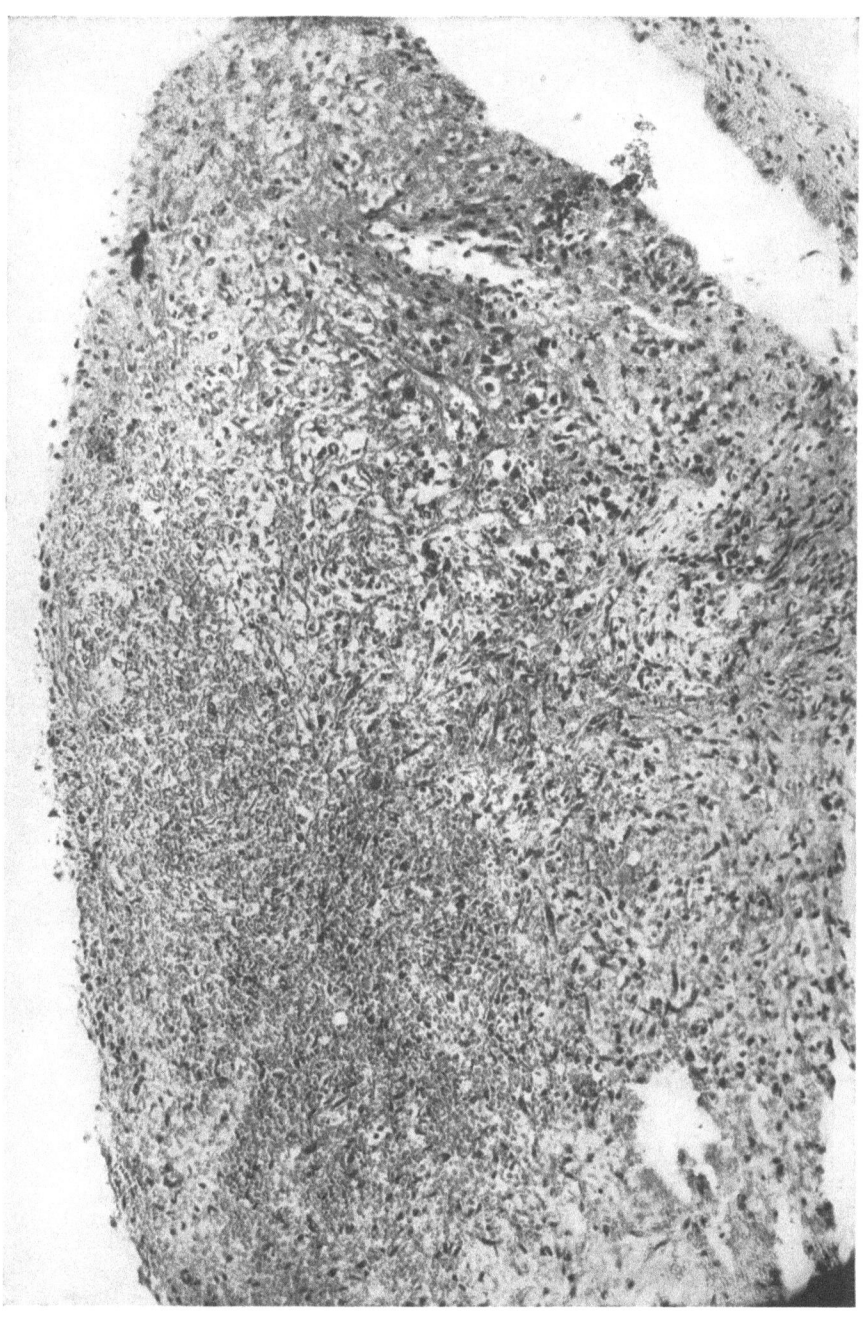

FIGURE 8. VACCINIA VALVULITIS. THE TRICUSPID VALVE IS GREATLY THICKENED BY LEUCOCYTIC INFILTRATION, HEMORRHAGE, AND FIBROBLASTIC PROLIFERATION
Hematoxylin and eosin. Magnification = × 140. (See note, Fig. 4.)

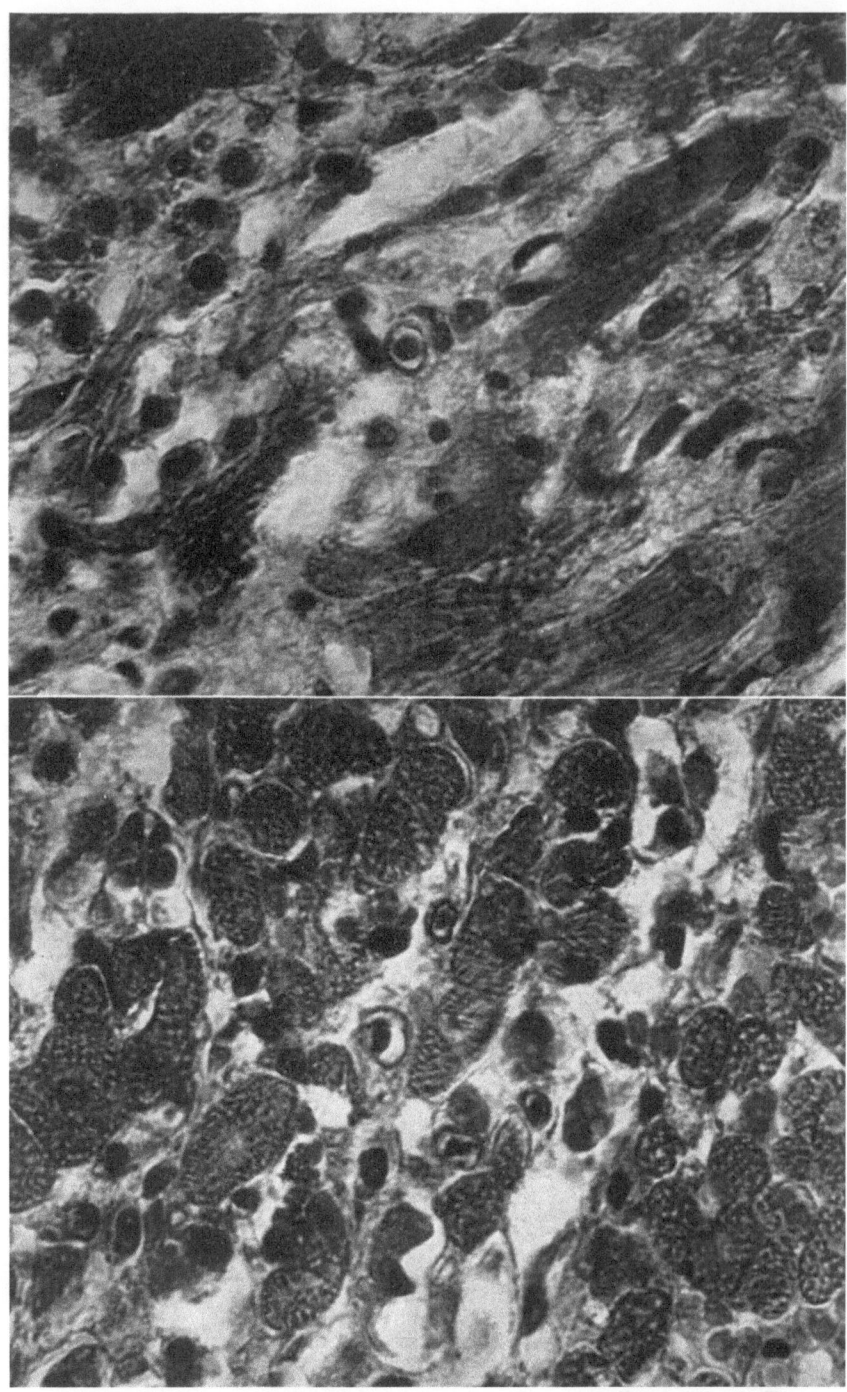

FIGURE 9. INTRANUCLEAR INCLUSION BODIES IN PSEUDORABIES MYOCARDITIS
Hematoxylin and eosin. Magnification = × 871. (See note, Fig. 4.)

variable as well. The lesion of vaccinia is an acute hemorrhagic necrosis with much leucocytic activity, while the effect of strain A fibroma is almost pure proliferation of fixed tissue with little or no inflammatory element. The other four excite reactions that can be classed at various points between these two extremes. Physically, the only criterion of differentiation is size. The vaccine and myxoma viruses are two of the largest filter passing agents that have been measured; the others of these six upon which determinations have been made are of varying smaller sizes.

All of these observations lead to the conclusion that the experiments described indicate most emphatically, in answer to the first question posed, that the ability of a virus to find lodgment in the heart and there produce morphological alterations is not a specific property of virus III nor of any group or class of viruses, but is, on the other hand, common to many and is dependent, not on the character of the virus but on the condition of the heart at the time when the virus in the circulating blood passes through it. Attention therefore was next turned to the second aspect of the problem.

FACTORS DETERMINING THE OCCURRENCE OF EXPERIMENTAL VIRAL CARDITIS

At first the only explanation that appeared to explain the cardiac localization of viral lesions was the somewhat indefinite concept of "overburdening" or "straining" the heart and thereby decreasing its resistance to virus in the blood stream. In all of the preceding experiments we had been struck by the fact that when acacia was used as the inducing agent, the myocardial lesions were predominantly right-sided and both auricle and ventricle were affected, but when pitressin was used, it was the left ventricle almost exclusively that suffered. This observation supported the overburdening idea, since the sudden addition of a large quantity of hypertonic solution of acacia to the venous blood might so increase its volume and thereby the venous blood pressure as to cause acute dilatation of the right auricle and ventricle and transient failure of the right side of the heart. Obviously, the sudden arteriolar spasm and elevation of arterial pressure that follow the intravenous injection of pitressin might have a similar effect on the left side. That this is not the true explanation was shown by two types of experiments. In one of these, measurements of the blood pres-

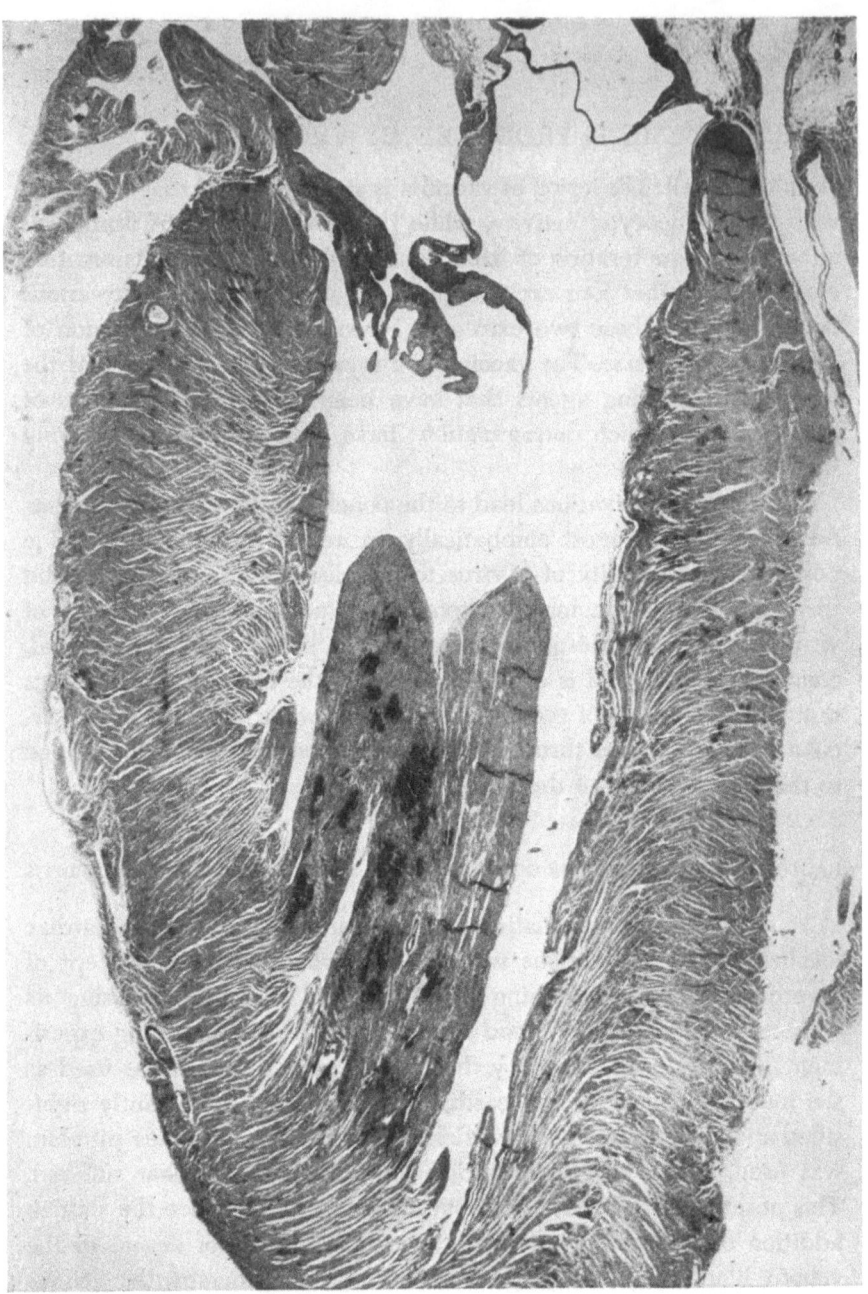

FIGURE 10. MYOCARDITIS AND VALVULITIS CAUSED BY THE INFLAMMATORY STRAIN OF THE FIBROMA VIRUS

Small foci of infiltration are scattered throughout the ventricular muscle, especially in the septum. In the papillary muscles there are large areas of necrosis and calcification. The mitral valve leaflets are markedly coarsened, thickened, and infiltrated as compared to the uninvolved aortic and tricuspid valves, which appear in the upper right-hand corner of the photograph. Hematoxylin and eosin. Magnification = $\times 75$.

sure of the right carotid artery and that of the marginal ear vein of the left ear were made and recorded by a kymograph before, during, and after the period in which acacia was injected into the marginal vein of the right ear of the rabbit. With the doses used in the virus work no significant alteration occurred in either pressure. In the other type of experiments, direct observations of the heart of the intact anesthetized animal were made while acacia was injected into the aural vein. No

TABLE 2

DATA ON RABBITS INOCULATED WITH VIRUS AND THEREAFTER SUBMITTED TO PROCEDURES TENDING TO CAUSE CARDIAC ANOXIA

Factors Causing Myocardial Anoxia	Rabbits Treated	RABBITS WITH CARDIAC LESIONS CAUSED BY VIRUS	
		Number	Percentage
Barium chloride*	5	5	100
Epinephrine hydrochloride*	7	6	85.7
Betahypophamine (pitressin)*	20	10	50
Acacia*	20	18	90

* Solutions of the substances were administered by intravenous injection.

dilatation of the right auricle and ventricle could be made out, but pallor of these chambers was striking during the period of the injection.

Since these negative results made it seem highly improbable that the "heart strain" hypothesis was valid as an explanation for the viral myocarditis, it was decided to submit animals to a variety of procedures designed to affect the heart in one way or another. Thus, in addition to betahypophamine (pitressin) solutions of epinephrine hydrochloride, barium chloride, digitalis, corn syrup, nikethamide ("coramine"), papaverine hydrochloride, and 0.85 percent sodium chloride were injected intravenously. The last was administered in 100 c.c. amounts as rapidly as the fluid could be forced from a syringe through a 20-gauge hollow needle. Another group of animals underwent chloroform narcosis.

The results fall into a definite pattern. Those procedures which reduce the supply of oxygen to the heart are followed by a high incidence and a high degree of severity of viral lesions of the heart. These have been placed in Table 2. Table 3 contains those procedures which are capable of damaging the heart or altering its function in a

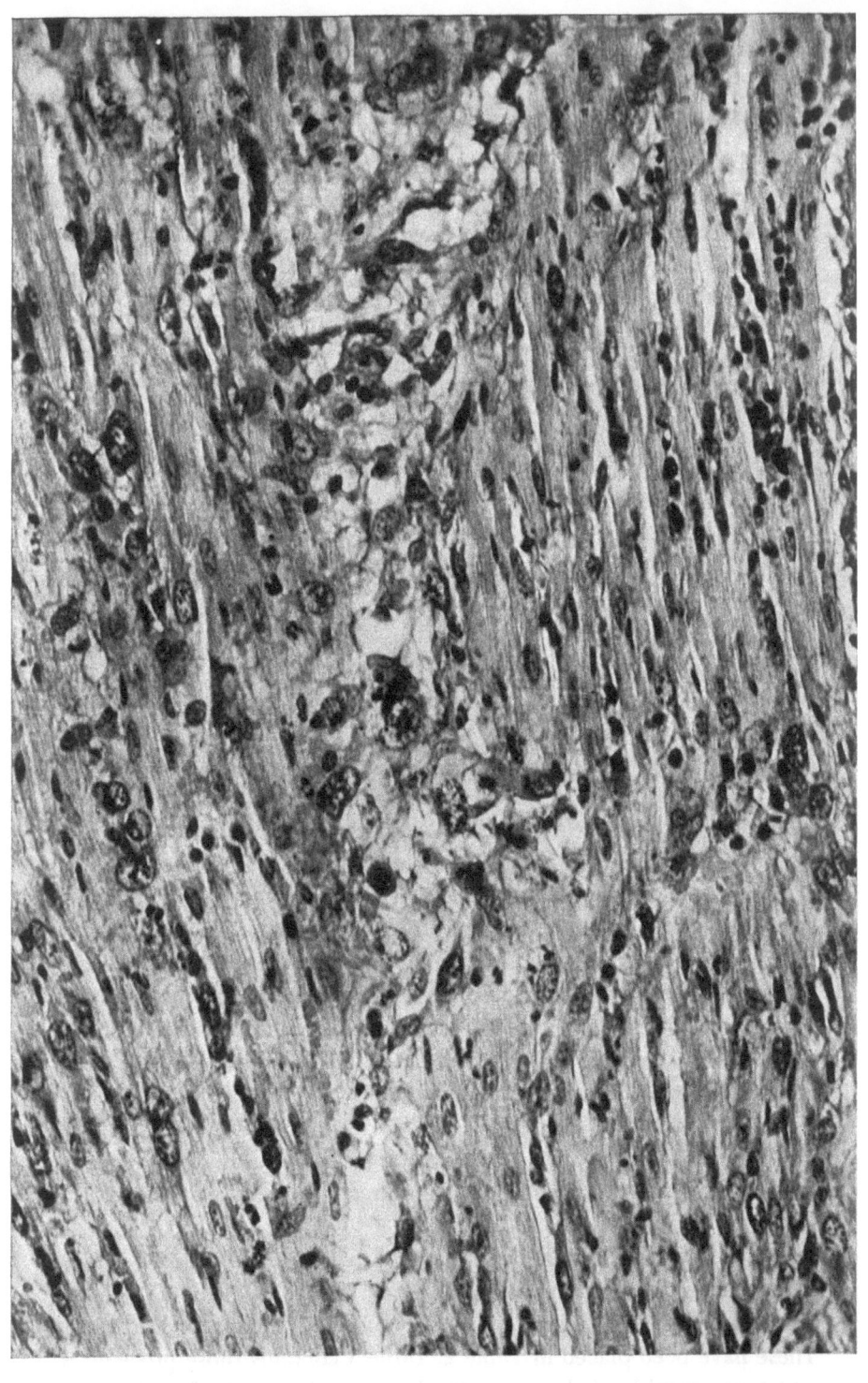

FIGURE 11. MYXOMA MYOCARDITIS. INFILTRATION AND REPLACEMENT OF HEART MUSCLE BY "MYXOMA CELLS"
Hematoxylin and eosin. Magnification = × 729.

variety of ways but which do not tend directly or indirectly to decrease the oxygen available to that organ.

The anatomic distribution of lesions between the two ventricles furnishes secondary evidence that a lack of oxygen is of importance in

TABLE 3

Data on Rabbits Inoculated with Virus and Thereafter Submitted to Procedures that May Affect the Heart But Do Not Cause Myocardial Anoxia

Factors Affecting Heart	Rabbits Treated	RABBITS WITH CARDIAC LESIONS CAUSED BY VIRUS	
		Number	Percentage
100 cc. of saline solution*	6	0	0
Corn syrup*	6	1	16.7
Nikethamide*	6	0	0
Digitalis*	6	0	0
Chloroform narcosis	6	1	16.7
Papaverine hydrochloride*	6	1	16.7
Controls: virus inoculations only	56	9	16.1

* Administered intravenously.

the development of viral lesions of the heart, since it is exactly the distribution of the areas to which the flow of oxygen is diminished by the different actions of acacia and the drugs constricting the coronary arteries. Thus, in the case of constriction of the coronary arteries, the right ventricle and the auricles are spared because the muscular walls of these chambers are so thin in the rabbit and contain so many endothelium-lined crevices communicating with the cavities that they are less dependent on coronary circulation and may receive a major part of their oxygen and nutriment directly from the blood within them. The thick left ventricle, however, is supplied by the blood flowing through the coronary arteries, and when that flow is diminished the muscle suffers. The inner portions of the myocardium and the plump papillary muscles of the left ventricle receive the terminal branches of the arteries and are therefore the regions most severely affected by the narrowing of the lumina of these vessels. This narrowing obviously may be brought about by the active contraction of the smooth muscle of the arterial walls that occurs under betahypophamine (3) or barium

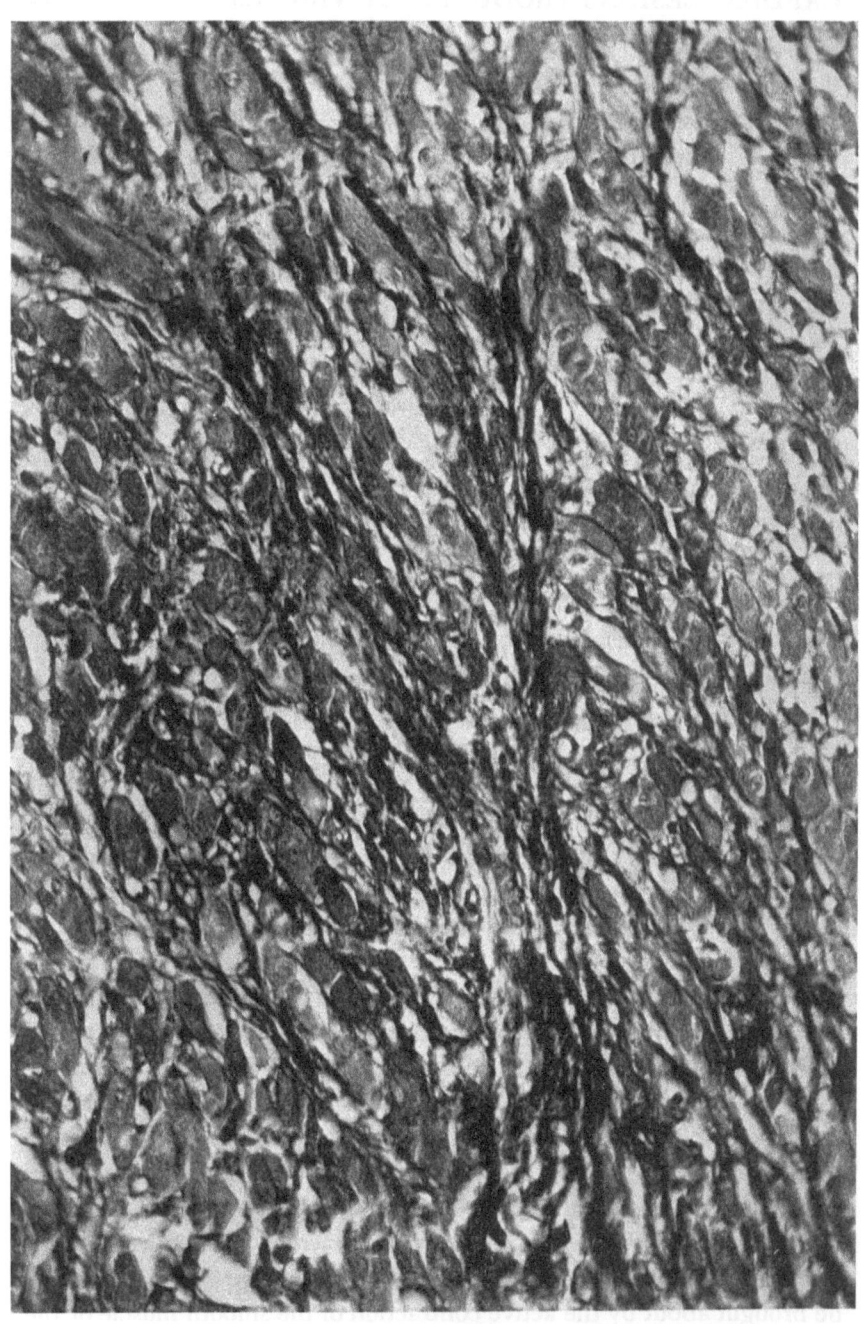

FIGURE 12. INTERSTITIAL FIBROSIS OF MYOCARDIUM IN FIBROMA-VIRUS INFECTION OF HEART
Masson's trichrome stain. Magnification = × 122.

chloride stimulation (4); or it may result from the great increase in the intramyocardial pressure that occurs, as well as the increase in intracardiac pressure, during the period of increased contractile force and acceleration of rate, brought about by epinephrine (5). The elevation of arterial blood pressure that follows the administration of all three substances also causes the intramyocardial pressure to rise. *In vivo* experiments conducted by Johnson and Di Palma (6) have demonstrated that during systole the intramyocardial pressure of the left ventricle exceeds the intra-aortic and hence the intracoronary pressure. The coronary arteries are thereby compressed, and the volume of blood flowing through them to the inner part of the myocardium and the papillary muscles is diminished. As was indicated earlier by Anrep and his associates (7), in strongly beating hearts the volume of blood flowing through even the more superficial arteries is reduced by the increase of intramyocardial pressure brought about by the stronger contraction.

The entirely different mechanism by which acacia produces cardiac anoxia explains why the lesions are predominantly on the right side of the heart when an intravenous injection of this substance is combined with the inoculation of virus. The acacia interferes with the interchange of oxygen between the hemoglobin of the red blood cells and the surrounding fluids and tissues. This action has been well demonstrated by Christie, Phatak, and Olney and others (8) and has been used to explain the cases of accidental death that followed the use of this substance as a plasma substitute some years ago. The greatest dilution of blood and hence the greatest interference with the passing of oxygen from red blood cell to tissue fluid occurs in the right auricle and ventricle as the acacia pours in from the injection site, the marginal vein of the ear, through the superior vena cava. Not only is the blood reaching the left ventricle more highly oxygenated after passing through the lungs, but also the mixture of blood of the superior and inferior venae cavae has become more complete, has decreased the local concentration of acacia, and has thereby diminished the interference with gaseous interchange.

Regardless of how convincing is the interpretation of the results of these experiments on the basis of cardiac anoxia or hypoxia, it rests on indirect evidence. Therefore the validity of the hypothesis was tested by inoculating animals with virus III and immediately thereafter placing them in an atmosphere deficient in oxygen. Figure 13 illustrates the apparatus used for this procedure. The oxygen in a sealed bell jar containing the rabbit was replaced to a variable extent

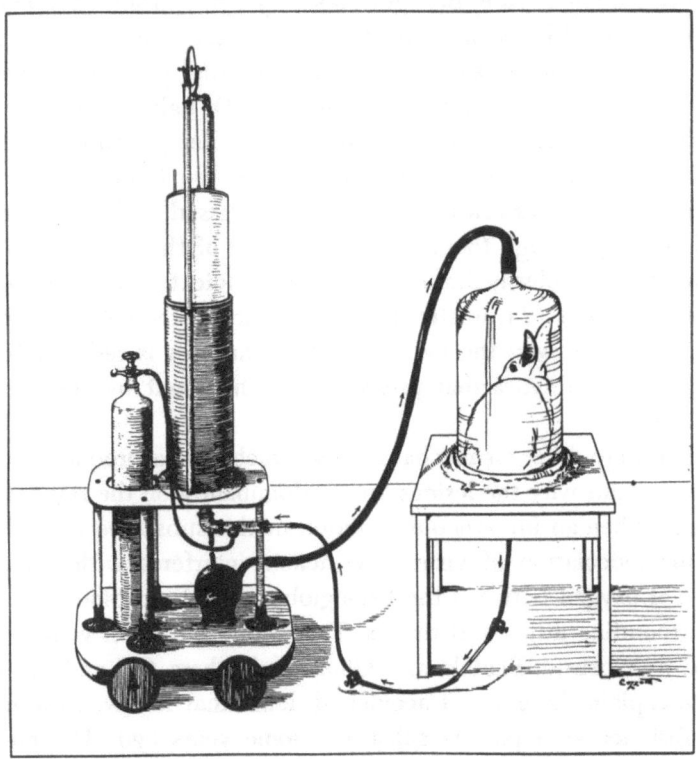

FIGURE 13. APPARATUS COMBINING A BELL JAR SEALED WITH "PLASTICINE," A SPIROMETER, AND A NITROGEN CYLINDER, BY WHICH RABBITS WERE SUBJECTED TO AN ATMOSPHERE DEFICIENT IN OXYGEN (See note, Fig. 4.)

by nitrogen, and the exhaled carbon dioxide and water was absorbed by soda lime in the spirometer which kept the gases circulating. The results of these experiments are comparable with those in which acacia, epinephrine, barium chloride, or pitressin had been used. The incidence of cardiac inflammation was 66.7 percent; twelve out of eighteen experimental animals developed lesions, but the individual lesions tended to be less severe.

To draw a closer parallel to human heart disease, especially to rheumatic fever, a final study was embarked upon in an attempt to show at least one functional alteration accompanying the structural changes of this experimental acute myocarditis.

Doctor Harold Levine (9) participated in this phase of the work by recording and interpreting electrocardiographic tracings made on twenty-five rabbits during the course of virus III myocarditis. In all but three he discovered definite abnormalities in cardiac function, including complete auriculoventricular heart block during the period in which acute myocarditis existed. It was to some extent possible to correlate the electrocardiographic abnormalities with anatomical lesions.

THE SIGNIFICANCE OF EXPERIMENTAL VIRAL CARDITIS IN SPONTANEOUS DISEASE

The similarity in morphology of the "pancarditis" that can be produced by experimental viral infection to human rheumatic heart disease and to other inflammations of unknown etiology suggests again, in spite of evidence to the contrary, that these lesions too may be of viral origin. Repeated attempts have been made in many laboratories to recover a virus by means of animal inoculation from the tissues and fluids of individuals suffering from rheumatic fever. The fact that none of these has had any convincing success does not preclude the possibility of viral etiology, since, as is well known, there are viruses of men and animals that are quite host-specific and ordinarily produce disease in only one species. In man perhaps varicella is the best example, since the viral origin of this less serious disease is substantiated by transmission experiments in children and by the morphological evidence provided by the intranuclear inclusion bodies in the lesions. Virus III holds an exactly similar position in relation to the rabbit.

Cases of myocarditis in man proven to be of viral origin by isolation of the agent from the heart have not come to my attention. On the other hand, there are a multitude of instances in which it is altogether probable that a virus brought about the inflammation of the heart. One of the most convincing reports is that of Finland, Parker, Barnes, and Joliffe (10), in which they describe an acute nonbacterial myocarditis occurring during the course of fatal influenza A pneumonia in which the virus was isolated from the lungs. The literature of electrocardiography is filled with reports of cases of myocarditis complicating influenza, measles, mumps, and other viral diseases in which the diagnosis was made by the tracing in patients who later recovered.

Saphir (11) has recently reviewed 240 cases of myocarditis of unknown but nonbacterial cause, variously designated as "isolated," "primary interstitial," "idiopathic," or "Fiedler's myocarditis." It seems likely, judging from illustration and description, that in a fair proportion of these the etiologic factor may have been a virus of one sort or another. The occurrence of so many cases in children supports this view. One obvious reason for the absence of instances in which a virus has been isolated from hearts such as these is purely technical: the pathologist is not "set up" for the necessary procedure. Another is the fact that the nature of the disease process is not suspected until the microscopic sections are examined.

Evidence that a spontaneous myocarditis does occur is furnished by Helwig and Schmidt (12), who recovered a virus, from two chimpanzees dying of congestive heart failure, that is capable of causing myocarditis not only in the ape but in guinea pigs and rabbits as well.

In conclusion and summary, then, it seems fairly well established that the heart of the rabbit can be infected by viruses of several quite different varieties and that when the virus is the sort that calls forth an acute inflammatory type of response all parts of the heart—pericardium, muscle, endocardium, and valves—may be involved. These lesions have a striking similarity to those of rheumatic carditis in man. The lodging and multiplication of the virus in the heart are greatly facilitated and the severity of the lesions there is enhanced if the oxygen supplied to that organ is drastically reduced in amount in the initial period of infection.

REFERENCES

1. Nedzel, A. J., Experimental endocarditis, *Arch. Path.*, 1937, 24:143.
2. Clark, P. F., and P. E. Svec, Experimental subacute bacterial endocarditis, *J. Bact.*, 1938, 35:55.
3. (a) Clark, G. A.: Action of posterior pituitary pressor extract on rabbit's vascular system, *J. Physiol.*, 1929, 68:166. (b) Essex, H. E., R. G. E. Wegria, J. F. Herrick, and F. C. Mann, Effect of certain drugs on coronary blood flow of trained dog. *Am. Heart J.*, 1940, 19:554. (c) Sollmann, T., *A Manual of Pharmacology*, p. 459 (Philadelphia, 1942).
4. Sollman, T., *A Manual of Pharmacology*, p. 554 (Philadelphia, 1942).

5. Goodman, L., and A. Gilman, *The Pharmacological Basis of Therapeutics*, p. 403 (New York, 1941).
6. Johnson, J. R., and J. R. Di Palma, Intramyocardial pressure and its relation to aortic blood pressure, *Am. J. Physiol.*, 1939, 125:234.
7. Anrep, G. V., E. W. H. Cruickshank, A. C. Downing, and A. Subba Rau, Coronary circulation in relation to cardiac cycle, *Heart*, 1927, 14:111. Anrep, G. V., and H. Hausler, Coronary circulation: effect of changes of blood-pressure and of output of heart, *J. Physiol.*, 1928, 65:357. Anrep, G. V., J. C. Davis, and E. Volhard, Effect of pulse pressure upon coronary blood flow, *Ibid.*, 1931, 73:405. Anrep, G. V., and E. von Saalfedd, Effect of cardiac contraction upon coronary flow, *Ibid.*, 1933, 79:317.
8. Christie, A., N. M. Phatak, and M. B. Olney, Effect of intravenous acacia on physio-chemical properties of blood, *Proc. Soc. Exp. Biol. & Med.*, 1935, 32:670. Studdiford, W. E., Severe and fatal reactions following intravenous use of gum acacia glucose infusions, *Surg., Gynec. & Obst.*, 1937, 64:772.
9. Pearce, J. M., and H. D. Levine, The anatomic cause of electrocardiographic changes in virus myocarditis of rabbits, *Am. Heart. J.*, 1943, 25:102.
10. Finland, M., F. Parker, Jr., M. W. Barnes, and L. S. Joliffe, Acute myocarditis in influenza A infections, two cases of non-bacterial myocarditis, with isolation of virus from the lungs, *Am. J. Med. Sci.*, 1945, 209:455.
11. Saphir, O.: Myocarditis: a general review, with an analysis of two hundred and forty cases, *Arch. Path.*, 1941, 32:1000; 1942, 33:88.
12. Helwig, F. C., and E. C. H. Schmidt, A filter-passing agent producing interstitial myocarditis in anthropoid apes and small animals. *Science*, 1945, 102:31.

Chapter 10

PATHOLOGY OF YELLOW FEVER

By J. E. Ash, *Former Scientific Director, American Registry of Pathology, Army Institute of Pathology,* Washington, D. C.

LITTLE CAN BE ADDED to the story of the morphologic changes in yellow fever as described by the pioneers Councilman (1), Torres (2), Klotz (3), and Cowdry (4). From a study of the relatively considerable material in the files of the Army Institute of Pathology, it is easy to confirm the classic features described by these gentlemen, and equally easy to conclude that the only specific diagnostic features are the type of liver damage and the Councilman hyaline degeneration. The changes in the other organs that were once considered very suggestive, if not diagnostic, have proved to be nonspecific after comparison with those caused by other infections. These include such details as "calcium casts," hyaline necrosis of malpighian corpuscles of the spleen, and the large basophilic macrophages in spleen, lymph nodes, and bone marrow. As a matter of fact, even the Councilman body is mimicked in other forms of liver necrosis. There is no disease, however, that produces such a "jumbled necrosis" of the liver as does yellow fever. One can be reasonably certain of the diagnosis, even with a low-power survey of the yellow-fever liver. In the early stages necrosis may be spotty (salt and pepper necrosis) or diffuse, but in either case it affects the cells of the midzones, locations readily identified by the intact cells about the portal areas and the central veins.

It is not necessary to repeat the minutiae of the morphologic changes in yellow fever because they have already been painstakingly described, but I shall review them briefly for purposes of orientation before attempting an interpretation of the pathology.

The cadaver may show residual jaundice emphasized by the pallor resulting from the hemorrhages characteristic of the disease clinically. These are most prominent in the gastro-intestinal tract, in the subepicardium, particularly the posterior portion, near the auriculoventricular junction, beneath the pleura, in the lungs, and, less frequently, in

* Now the Armed Forces Institute of Pathology.

PATHOLOGY OF YELLOW FEVER

the urinary bladder. Cutaneous hemorrhages are not so common as in the rickettsial diseases. An almost constant finding is the coffee-grounds content of the stomach. The urine may be dark red.

The liver grossly is very deceiving. While it may be slightly enlarged and less firm than normal, with an increase in the yellowish tone of the cut surface, it is not possible to judge from gross examination the extent of parenchymal damage.

The spleen may be moderately enlarged and somewhat softer than normal.

The kidneys are generally swollen, the parenchyma is pale, and congestion is apparent, particularly in the medulla.

Gross changes of the central nervous system are minimal; they are limited to congestion and possible petechiae, most common in the pons and medulla.

MICROSCOPIC CHANGES

Liver. The details of the hepatic changes vary considerably with the stage of the disease in which the patient died, the time elapsed after death before fixation of tissues, and the type of fixation. These factors particularly affect the recognition of the nuclear inclusion bodies.

Fatty degeneration is always present but varies greatly in extent, with the fat appearing as both fine and large globules. Hyaline degeneration takes place not only in the frankly damaged cells of the midzones but also in the less involved cells of the peripheral and central areas. According to Klotz, so long as the change is only fatty degeneration and cloudy swelling, even when the nuclei are hydropic, the process is not irreversible. The presence of the hyalin, however, indicates that the cell will die. At first there are only hyaline particles; they eventually coalesce, become more and more compact, and shrink sufficiently within the cell to produce a slight fissure of separation from the remaining cytoplasm. The Councilman bodies are usually rounded, and in spite of their hyaline character they practically always show varying numbers of minute vacuoles, fine cracks, and some granularity. They range from 5 to 25 microns in diameter. A common finding is a pyknotic crescent-shaped nucleus attached to one portion of the periphery. As a matter of fact, if there is difficulty in locating typical Councilman bodies, this darkly staining nuclear crescent may be utilized under the lower power as a "tracer." The bodies may be present in cells with relatively intact nuclei, or the cells may become entirely necrotic, rupture, and liberate the hyaline bodies. They may be seen, therefore, either free in the parenchymal meshwork or in the sinusoids. The Councilman bodies are readily distinguishable from the hyaline structures characteristic of alcoholic cirrhosis which Mallory described. The latter are not so readily demonstrable; they tend to be branched and to surround the cell nucleus and are not vacuolated. As was originally stated by Councilman, masses simulating Councilman bodies can be seen in other types of liver necrosis—in carbon-tetrachloride poisoning, for example. Some of these are obviously inspissated bile, either still in a bile capillary or free as the result of necrosis of the surrounding liver cells. Although at times they may have a granular appearance, they do not have the fine vacuoles or fissures seen in the Councilman bodies.

The nuclear changes are interesting but variable, and while Cowdry insisted that the inclusions in yellow fever have characteristics that distinguish them from other nuclear inclusions, these are difficult to appreciate in run-of-the-mill material. Nuclear inclusions are not so commonly seen in human material as in monkeys with experimental infections. The inclusions are acidophilic and first appear as discrete clumps, which increase in size through conglutination. They may assume a variety of shapes, crescent, so-called "butterfly of Torres," or they may be present as multiple clumps. The chromatin of the nucleus tends to collect on the nuclear membrane. The nucleolus may maintain its central position or migrate to the periphery. It becomes paler and may finally take an acidophilic stain, when it may be confused with the inclusion bodies; however, it is more homogeneous and hyaline than the latter. The acidophilic inclusions are supposed to be more numerous in the early stages of the disease when the virus is still present in the blood. They represent, according to Cowdry, an oxychromatic degeneration of nucleoplasm.

Independent of the inclusions, the nuclei of the parenchymal cells undergoing degeneration and necrosis may suffer the so-called explosion karyorrhexis of Klotz, that is, rupture of the nucleus-liberating chromatin masses; or by process of lysis the nucleus may greatly enlarge, become vacuolated, and finally be seen as a thin-walled sac free of nuclear material, the so-called empty nucleus. Mitosis is very rare but may be simulated by the rearrangement of chromatin during the process of disintegration. These changes make the nuclei particularly prominent in the microscopic field.

The cytoplasm of the cells may show a varying number of bright ocher granular bodies, which Villela (5) interprets as the result of impregnation of disintegrating Councilman bodies with bile pigment. He regards them as diagnostic evidence of yellow fever even in the absence of the classic Councilman bodies. They may also be found free among nonnecrotic parenchymal cells but are found more frequently within macrophages and Kupffer cells.

The Kupffer cells are usually badly damaged, greatly enlarged, and vacuolated; at times they contain pigment particles but never the hyaline particles of the Councilman degeneration.

Ordinarily there is little damage to the reticulum framework of the lobule, but intralobular hemorrhages are not unknown. Exudate is not a feature of the reaction, although mononuclear cells and a few polymorphonuclear leucocytes may be found in the necrotic zones. One detail in the picture is similar to that seen in epidemic hepatitis and other forms of liver necrosis, that is, the presence of large numbers of macrophages loaded with prominently eosinophilic globules of hyaline debris.

Kidney. While the kidney is invariably damaged and seriously so, the changes cannot be considered specific. Fatty degeneration of the usual type is practically always present to some degree. Cloudy swelling and hyaline degeneration, particularly the latter, may be extreme, and masses of hyalin, indistinguishable from Councilman bodies, may be found in the tubular cells at all levels, or in the lumens of the lower tubules. The glomeruli ordinarily are not so severely affected, although there may be much intracapsular precipitate and, in other instances, agglutinates on the outer wall of the capsule. The hyaline material in the lower tubule may simulate blood very closely, but intratubular hemorrhage is not common, although congestion of the medullary vessels is frequently prominent and there may be hemorrhages. While calcific deposits are considered a classic feature, they were not outstanding in the material at the Institute, and it is believed that the so-called calcium casts are more frequently crystalline and laminated deposits of material other than calcium. The pathogenesis of the kidney lesions is debatable. There is little or no indication that the virus per se localizes in the kidney; nuclear inclusions are not found and there is a question whether the fatty and hyaline degenerations are not largely secondary to the rapid and serious liver damage (choline deficiency) or the result of the general toxic state.

Heart. Fatty degeneration of the muscle fibers may be striking, even to the extent that it may be grossly evident in the flabby condition of the organ; but there is little, if any, interstitial reaction. The heart differs remarkably in this respect from the heart in the rickettsial diseases, in which the interstitial reaction is intense and the damage to the muscle fibers minimal.

Intestines. There is always submucosal congestion and there may be frank hemorrhages. Varying amounts of a nonspecific interstitial exudate, predominantly mononuclear, are usually present in the submucosa.

Lungs. In the absence of secondary bacterial infection, the only feature—and it not always evident—is small hemorrhages, subpleural and deeper in the parenchyma.

Spleen. Striking changes are usually observed in the spleen, consisting most characteristically of diminution of lymphocytes in both the cell columns and the follicles, and the presence of large basophilic macrophages. These are not specific for yellow fever but are of the same nature as those seen in a variety of infections, particularly the rickettsial diseases and Oroya fever. In the follicles, in addition to the reduction in lymphocytes, there are commonly accumulations of macrophages which undergo colliquative hyaline necrosis, forming large amoeboid masses that are the most prominent histologic feature. These again are not specific for yellow fever, as they were considered by Klotz. The follicular arteries commonly show a pale hyaline swelling. Small hemorrhages may be present in the pulp.

Brain. While yellow fever virus is regarded as neurotropic and undoubtedly is when directly injected into the brain, in natural infections the normal blood-brain barrier seems to protect the central nervous system from damage except in young children, in whom frank encephalitis may develop. In adults the brain lesions are comparatively insignificant and certainly nonspecific. They consist of perivascular hemorrhage, most common in the hypothalamus but sometimes seen in the cerebral hemispheres and the cerebellum. Very occasionally there may be limited vascular cuffing of lymphocytes. There are practically no involvement of the nerve cells, no inclusion bodies, and no glial reaction (Stevenson [6]).

COMMENTS

The only really specific pathologic feature in yellow fever is the liver damage, and this raises the question as to the tropism of the causative virus. Is this, in fact, limited to the liver cells or is there a direct involvement of other organs, particularly the kidneys and the spleen? From a review of the literature and from the experience with material at the Institute it would seem that the primary, or at least predominant, specific localization is in the liver parenchyma. Certainly it seems to be established that Stevenson is correct in his conclusion that the virus in nature is not normally neurotropic.

The prominent parenchymal fatty degeneration, especially of the liver, kidneys, and heart muscle, is an incidental disturbance. The severe and characteristic hyaline degeneration of liver and kidneys suggests a common specific etiologic factor, and it is the only feature in the picture that indicates a direct influence of the virus on both liver and kidneys. It is the only element in the picture that can not be duplicated in tissues affected by other infections. Such severe kidney damage is not seen ordinarily in other types of liver necrosis. It cannot be a cholemic nephrosis because the jaundice is neither prolonged nor intense, and it would be difficult to explain entirely on the basis of the vague hepatorenal syndrome. In chloroform and carbon-tetrachloride poisonings the liver destruction is undoubtedly very rapid and may be extensive, but fatty degeneration is the prominent feature of the kidney damage. The same is true of the fulminant type of hepatitis, in which death occurs within ten days. Destruction of liver cells is rapid, and it may be total in the involved lobules, but Lucké and Mallory (7, 8) were unable to find renal changes indicative of the specific hepatorenal syndrome. The majority of cases studied by them showed renal damage chiefly limited to fatty degeneration. This they attributed to factors other than the liver damage. It would seem from all evidences, therefore, that there is a possibility of specific action on the renal epithelium by the virus, but it is by no means definitely established. The picture varies from case to case, and such incidentals as the crystalline and starch-like bodies in the tubules are found in other conditions, carbon-tetrachloride poisoning, for example (9).

The constant circulatory features are probably an evidence of shock. Specific vascular damage is not demonstrable.

As was already stated, the changes in the spleen are in no way specific; both the basophilic macrophages and the colliquative necrosis in the follicles are found in a variety of infections.

An interesting corollary is the comparison of the pathology of viral diseases with that of the rickettsial infections. The differences are explainable, in part, by the variation in tropisms. The viruses are more specifically limited to certain organs or tissues, while the rickettsiae have a common affinity for the reticulo-endothelium and the vascular endothelium with, of course, the exception of those of the Q diseases. There is much similarity, therefore, in the pathology of the various rickettsial diseases; in general the changes are diffuse rather than localized. The clinical pictures of the various rickettsial diseases also exhibit considerable similarity. Each of the viral diseases is a specific clinical entity, and the specific pathology is limited to a particular cell group. Rickettsial diseases are characterized by intense vascular damage and by mononuclear exudate; other changes are incidental. Viral diseases are characterized by the comparative absence of vascular damage, and the effect is primarily on epithelial tissues.

There are still several problems the experimentalist must solve, among them the definite tropism of the virus and the pathogenesis of the renal and circulatory lesions.

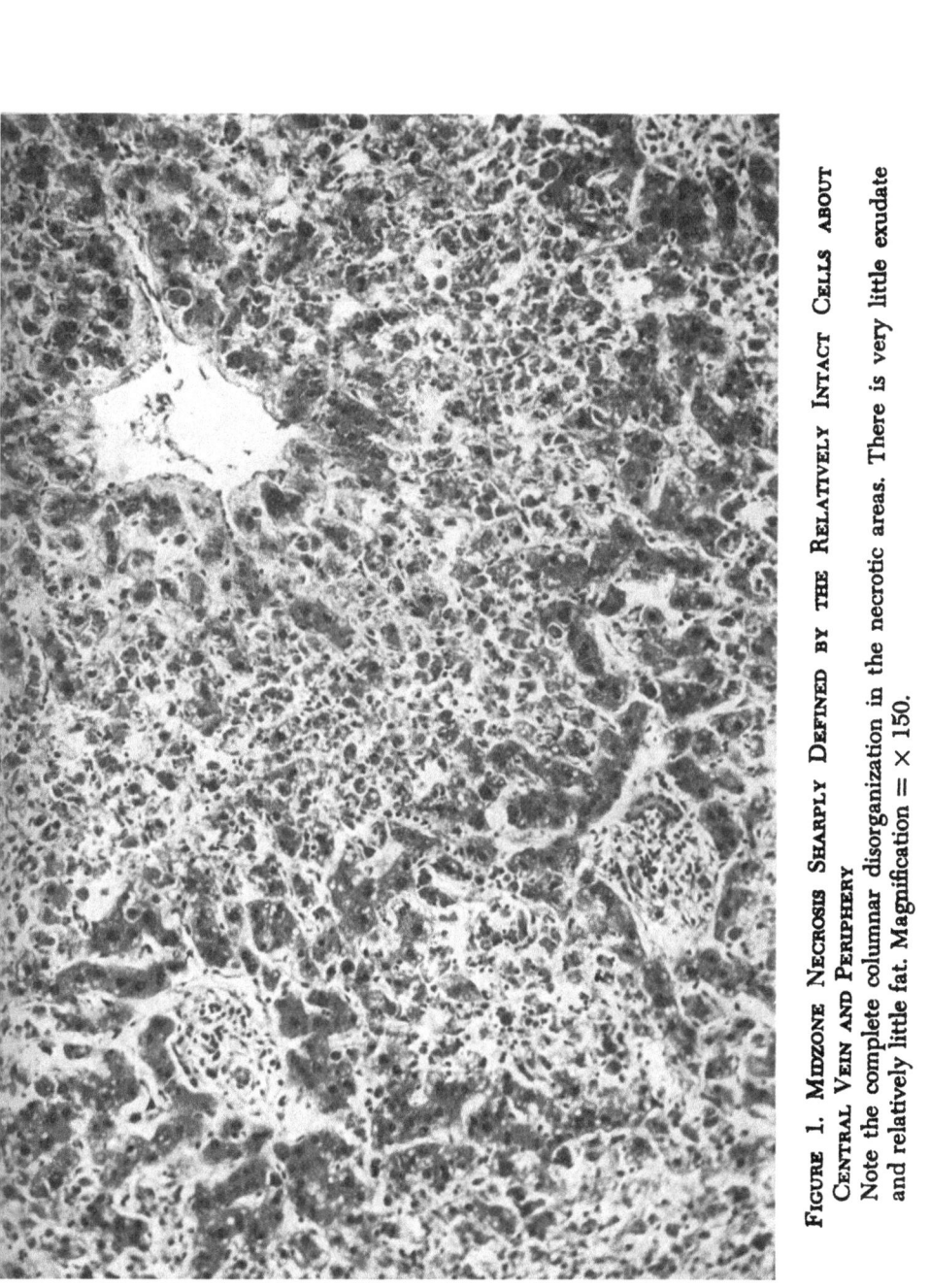

FIGURE 1. MIDZONE NECROSIS SHARPLY DEFINED BY THE RELATIVELY INTACT CELLS ABOUT CENTRAL VEIN AND PERIPHERY

Note the complete columnar disorganization in the necrotic areas. There is very little exudate and relatively little fat. Magnification = × 150.

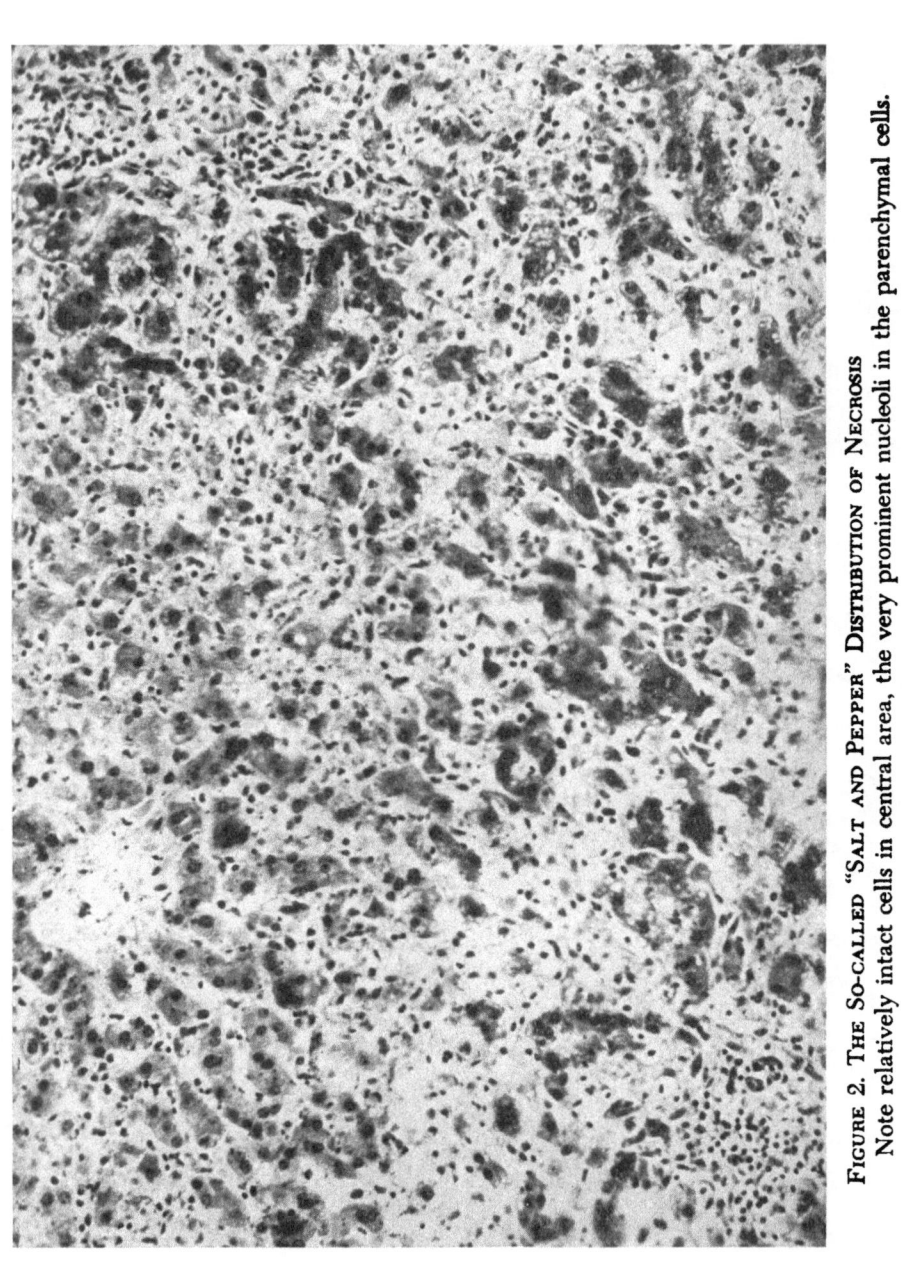

FIGURE 2. THE SO-CALLED "SALT AND PEPPER" DISTRIBUTION OF NECROSIS
Note relatively intact cells in central area, the very prominent nucleoli in the parenchymal cells.

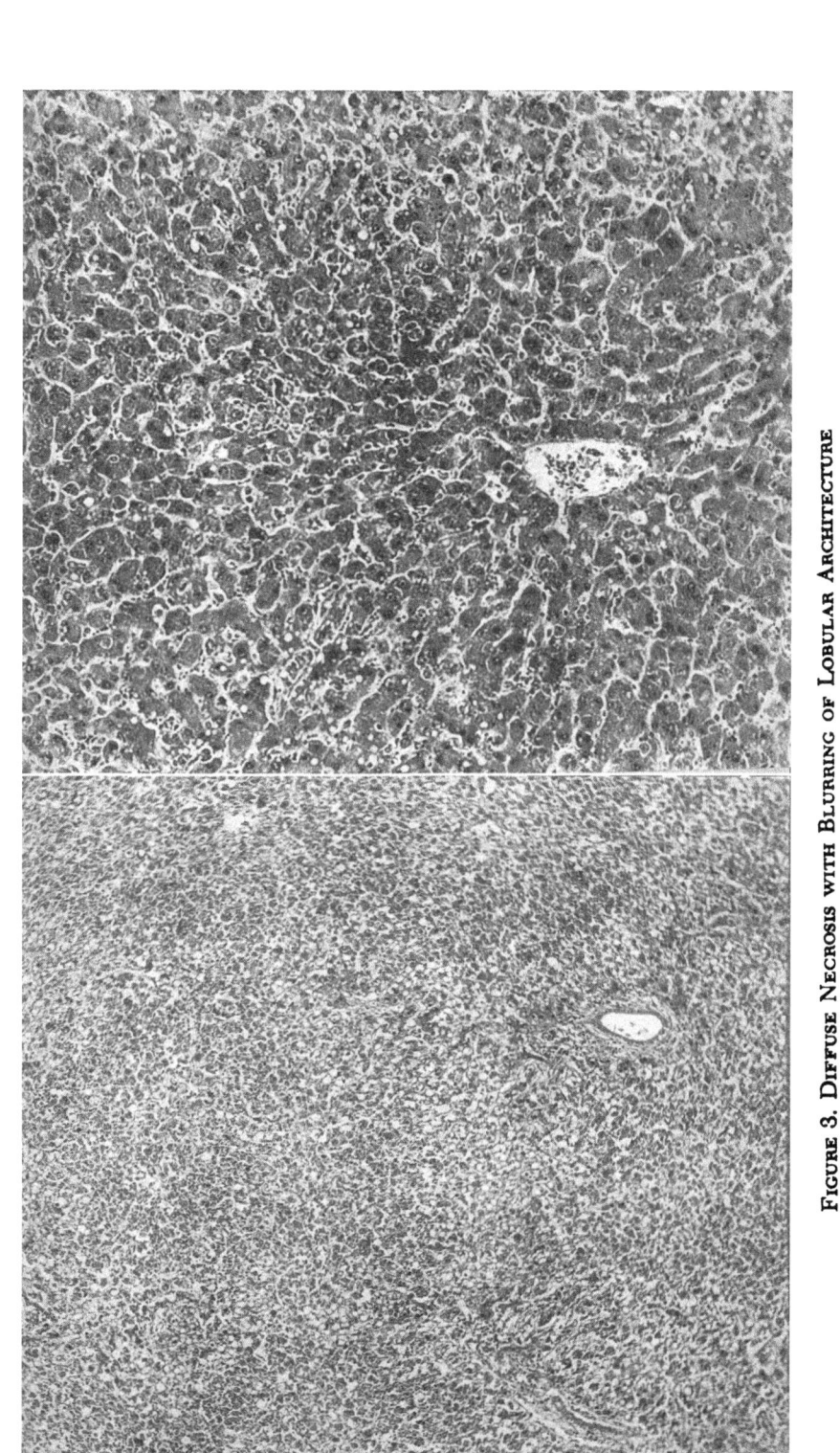

FIGURE 3. DIFFUSE NECROSIS WITH BLURRING OF LOBULAR ARCHITECTURE
Only a few relatively intact cells about the portal areas. Magnification = × 100.
FIGURE 4. NECROSIS MORE SUBTLE IN CHARACTER BUT MOST OBVIOUS IN MIDZONE
Relatively little fat. Magnification = × 114.

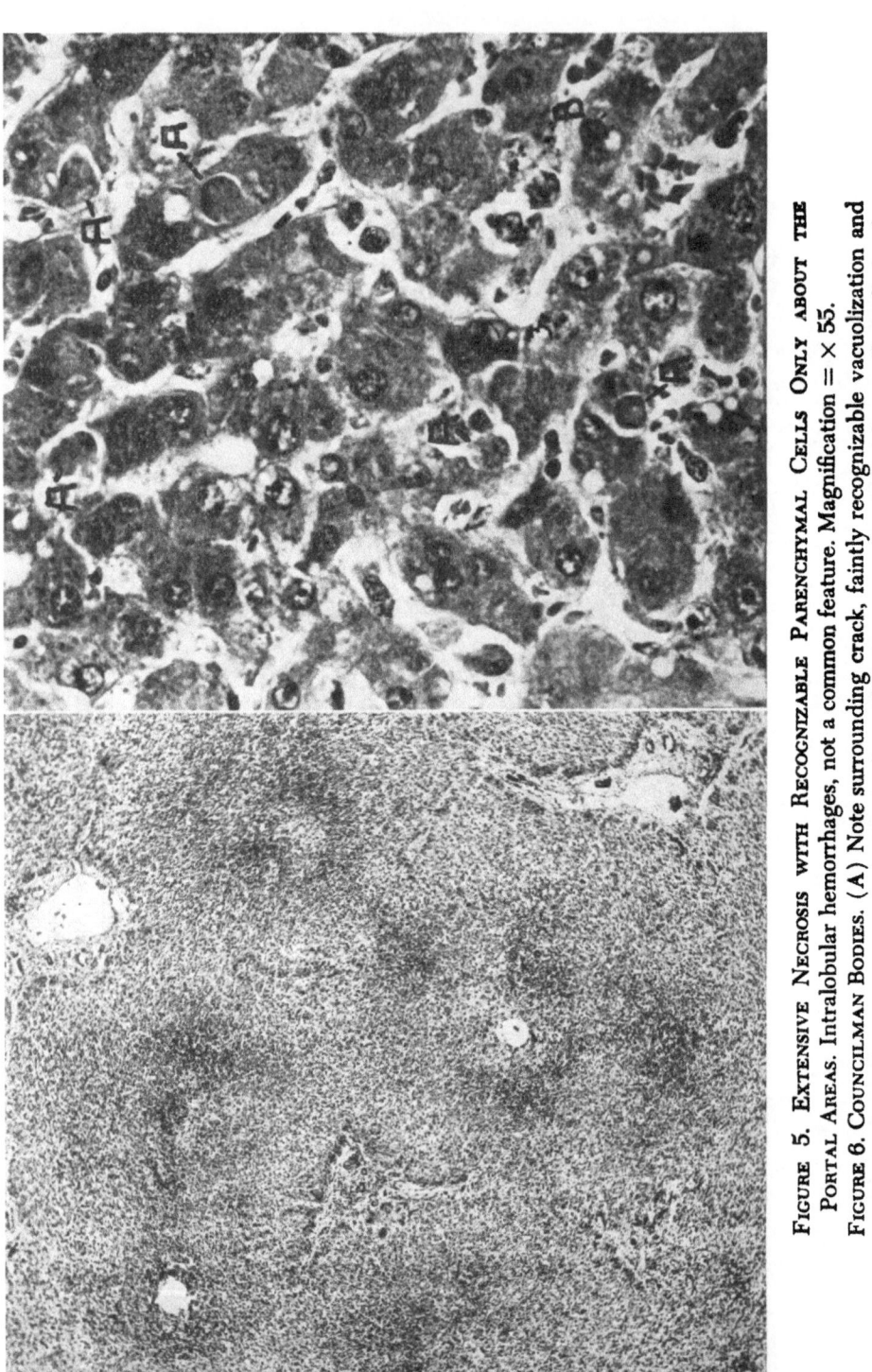

FIGURE 5. EXTENSIVE NECROSIS WITH RECOGNIZABLE PARENCHYMAL CELLS ONLY ABOUT THE PORTAL AREAS. Intralobular hemorrhages, not a common feature. Magnification = × 55.

FIGURE 6. COUNCILMAN BODIES. (A) Note surrounding crack, faintly recognizable vacuolization and lamination; (B) swollen vacuolated Kupffer cells. Note prominence of liver-cell nucleoli; the majority have migrated to the periphery. Magnification = × 450.

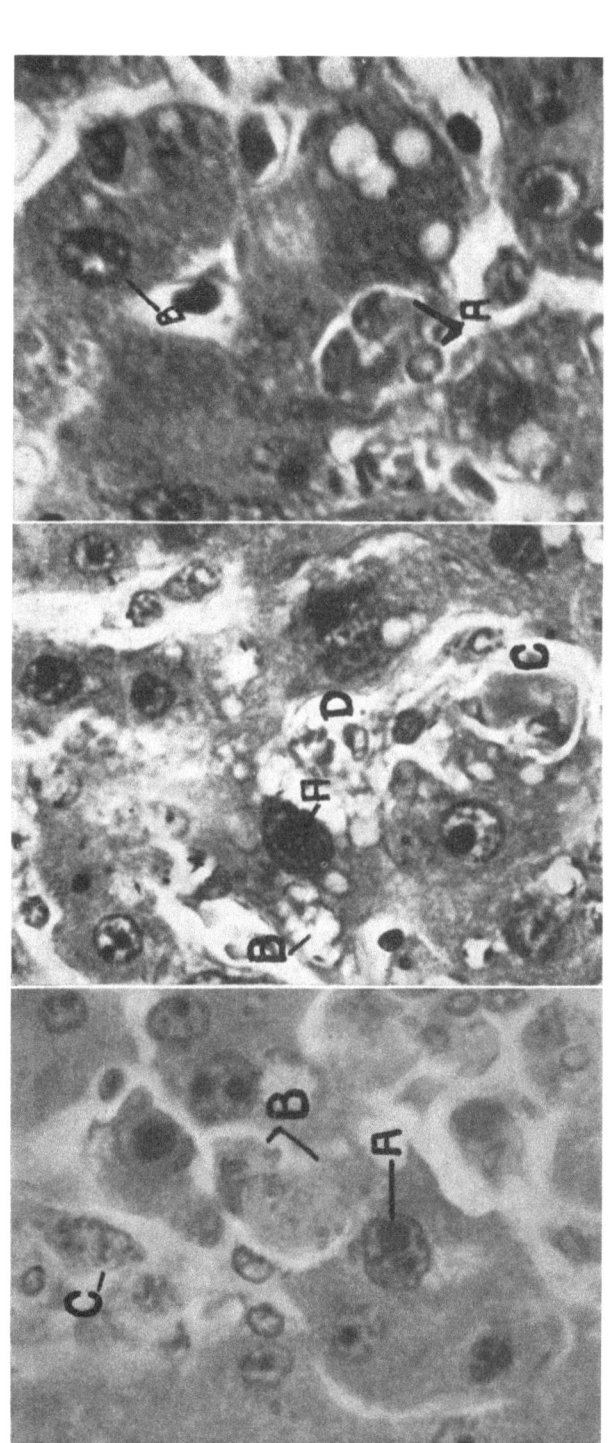

FIGURE 7. A. NUCLEAR INCLUSION. B. GRANULAR COUNCILMAN BODIES WITH NUCLEAR MATERIAL AT PERIPHERY. C. SWOLLEN, HYDROPIC KUPFFER CELLS
Magnification = × 755.
FIGURE 8. A. NUCLEOLUS UNDERGOING ACIDOPHILIC CHANGE. B. "EMPTY" NUCLEUS. C. COUNCILMAN BODY. D. "EXPLOSION" NUCLEUS
Magnification = × 705.
FIGURE 9. A. COUNCILMAN BODIES WITH NUCLEAR CRESCENT ATTACHED. B. MULTIPLE INTRANUCLEAR INCLUSIONS

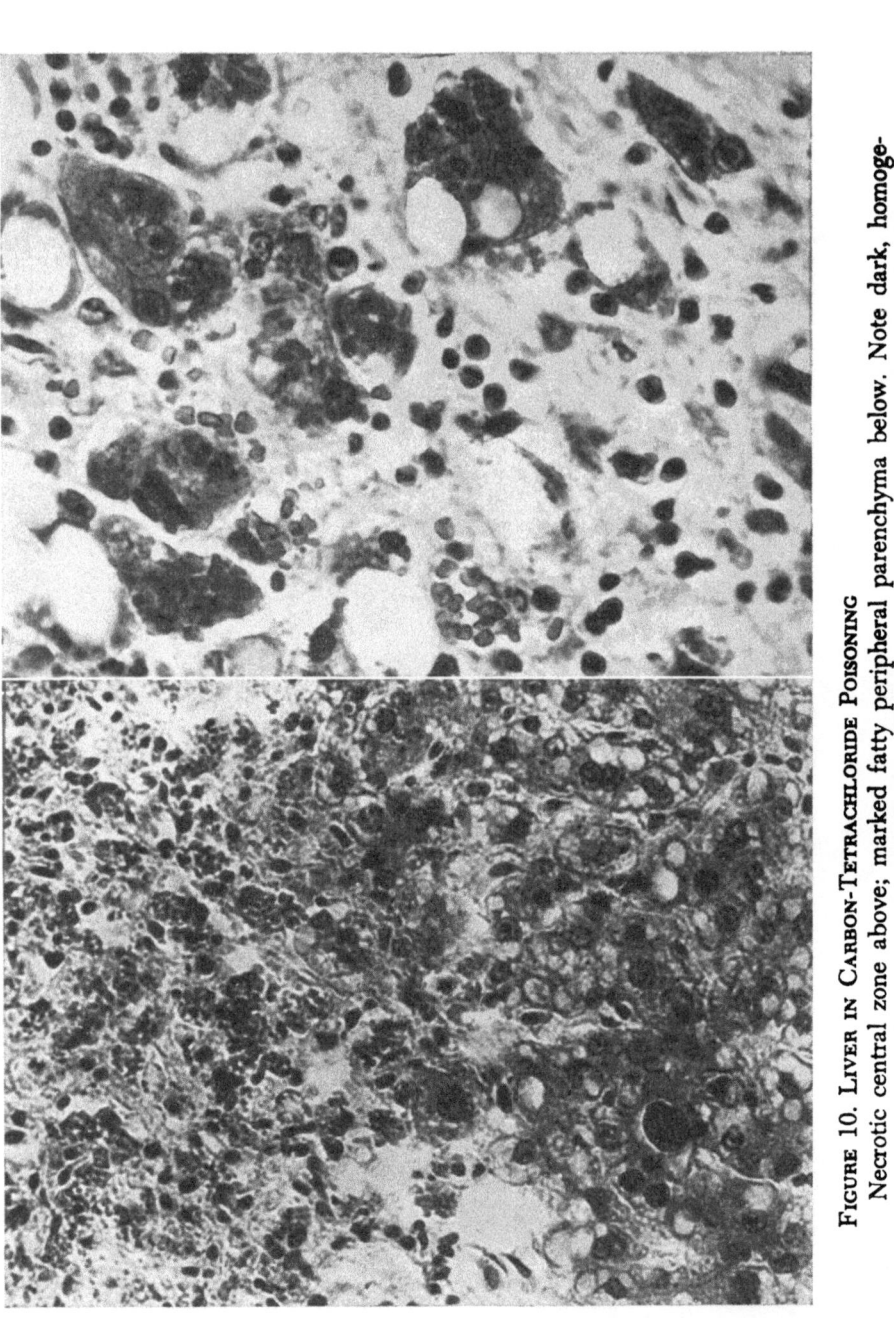

FIGURE 10. LIVER IN CARBON-TETRACHLORIDE POISONING
Necrotic central zone above; marked fatty peripheral parenchyma below. Note dark, homogeneous mass in latter with surrounding "crack" resembling Councilman body, actually bile cast. Magnification = × 305.

FIGURE 11. LIVER IN ALCOHOLIC CIRRHOSIS TO SHOW THE MALLORY HYALIN
It is branched, tends to surround nucleus. Magnification = × 600.

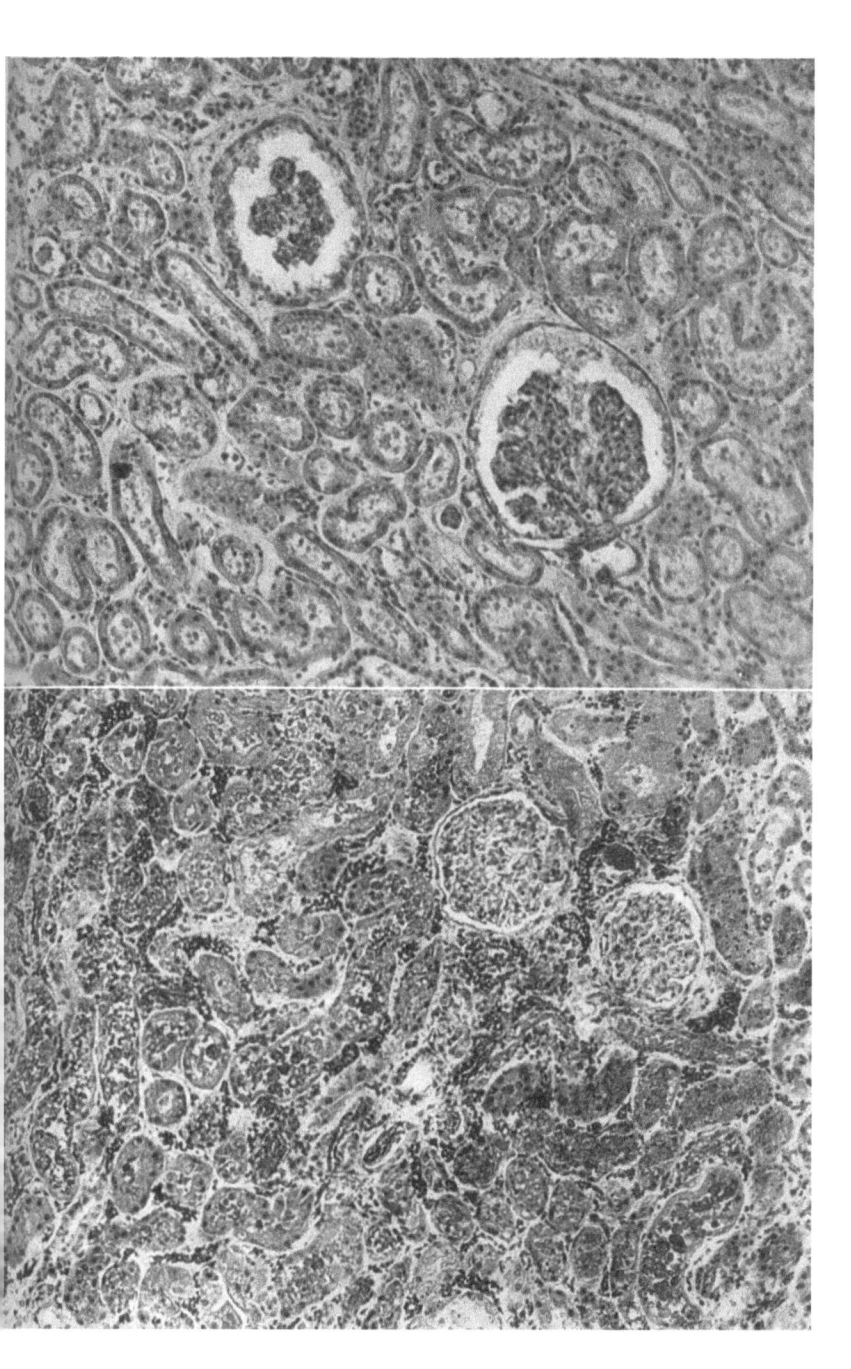

FIGURE 12. KIDNEY
Shows marked cloudy swelling, fatty and hyaline degeneration. Gross hyaline masses in lumina resembling Councilman bodies. Glomeruli relatively intact.
FIGURE 13. PRECIPITATE ON BOWMAN'S MEMBRANE; INTERSTITIAL EDEMA; THE LOW FORM OF EPITHELIAL DEGENERATION WITH NUMEROUS HYALINE BODIES
Magnification = × 114.

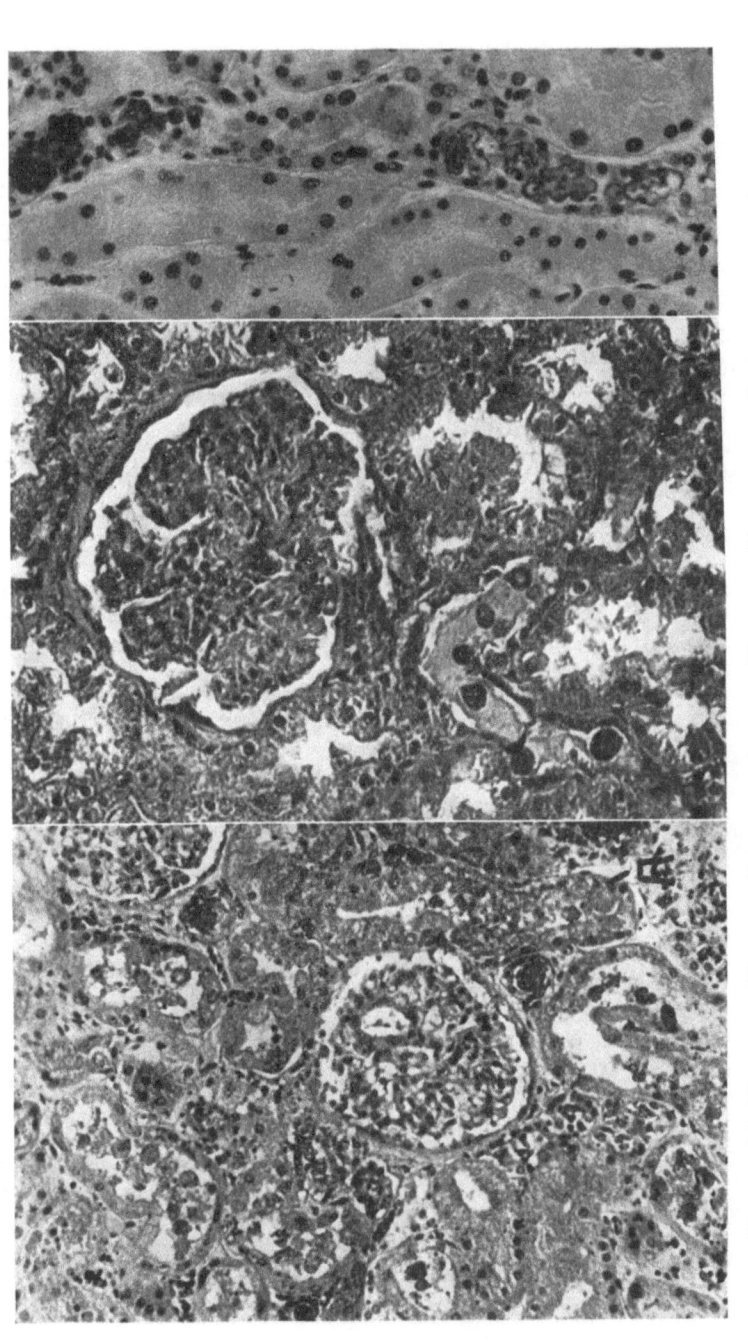

FIGURE 14. EXTREME HYALINE DEGENERATION OF TUBULAR EPITHELIUM, INTRACELLULAR COUNCILMAN-LIKE BODY AT A
A number of them in the tubular lumens. Magnification = × 180.
FIGURE 15. "LIME" CASTS, INCLUDING AMYLOID BODIES
FIGURE 16. "LIME" CASTS MADE UP OF NUMEROUS STARCH-LIKE BODIES

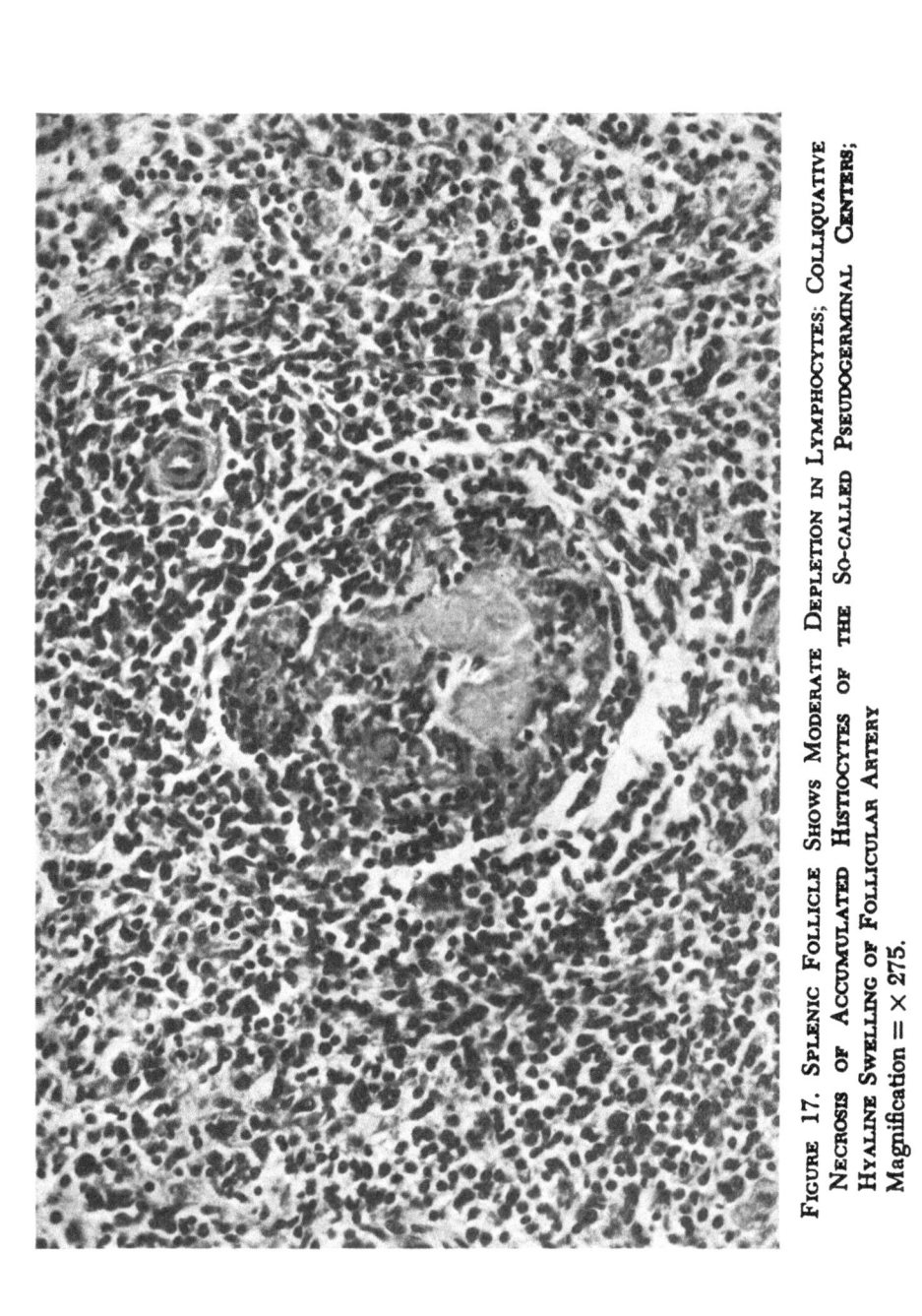

FIGURE 17. SPLENIC FOLLICLE SHOWS MODERATE DEPLETION IN LYMPHOCYTES; COLLIQUATIVE NECROSIS OF ACCUMULATED HISTIOCYTES OF THE SO-CALLED PSEUDOGERMINAL CENTERS; HYALINE SWELLING OF FOLLICULAR ARTERY
Magnification = × 275.

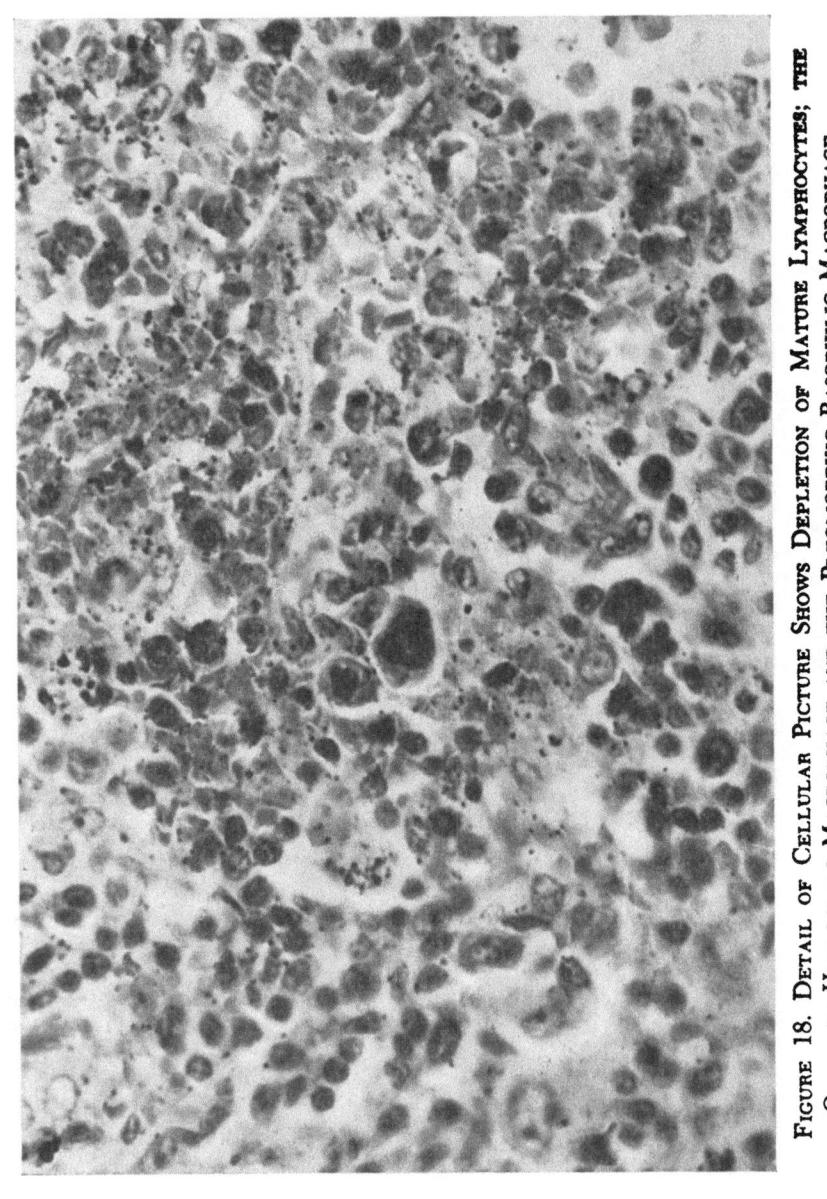

FIGURE 18. DETAIL OF CELLULAR PICTURE SHOWS DEPLETION OF MATURE LYMPHOCYTES; THE ORDINARY HISTIOCYTIC MACROPHAGE AND THE PLEOMORPHIC BASOPHILIC MACROPHAGE Magnification = × 640.

REFERENCES

1. Councilman, W. T., in G. M. Sternberg, *Report on the Etiology and Prevention of Yellow Fever*, Government Printing Office, Washington, D. C., 1890, p. 151.
2. Torres, C. M., Inclusions nucléaires acidophiles (dégénérescence oxychromatique) dans le foie de Macacus rhesus inoculé avec le virus brésilien de la fièvre jaune, *C. R. Soc. Biol.*, 1928, 99:1344.
3. Klotz, O., and T. H. Belt, The pathology of the spleen in yellow fever, *Am. J. Path.*, 1930, 6:655.
 ———, The pathology of the liver in yellow fever, *Am. J. Path.*, 1930, 6:663.
4. Cowdry, E. V., and S. F. Kitchen, Intranuclear inclusions in yellow fever, *Am. J. Hyg.*, 1930, 11:227.
5. Villela, E., Histology of human yellow fever when death is delayed, *Arch. Path.*, 1941, 31:665.
6. Stevenson, L. D., Pathologic changes in the nervous system in yellow fever, *Arch. Path.*, 1939, 27:249.
7. Lucké, B., The pathology of fatal epidemic hepatitis, *Am. J. Path.*, 1944, 20:471.
8. Lucké, B., and T. B. Mallory, The fulminant form of epidemic hepatitis, *Am. J. Path.*, 1946, 22:867.
9. Smetana, H., Nephrosis due to carbon tetrachloride, *Arch. Int. Med.*, 1939, 63:760.

Chapter 11

REACTIONS OF THE CELLS OF THE RESPIRATORY TRACT TO VIRUS INFECTIONS

BY THOMAS P. MAGILL, *Department of Microbiology and Immunology, Long Island College of Medicine*

IDEAS concerning the usefulness of histological methods in the identification of disease entities have changed somewhat during recent years; but whereas the pathologist of the past expected too much of such methods, the virologist of the present goes to the other extreme and, perhaps, expects too little. There is good reason, however, for the virologist's pessimism.

Virus infections differ from most bacterial infections in that the activity is essentially within the cell; and, obviously, there is a limit to the number of ways in which a cell may react. The inclusion body was the first of the cellular reactions to virus infection (or, perhaps, reaction of the virus to the cell) recognized by pathologists; for a time it was thought that such bodies were characteristic of virus infection, but it is now recognized that many, if not most, virus infections are not associated with typical inclusion bodies. Inflammatory processes are relegated to a secondary role.

Rivers (1) observes that the primary reaction of cells to virus infections must be proliferative, degenerative, or a combination of those two processes. In some of the less acute virus infections there is sufficient time for the combined proliferative and degenerative processes to form a recognizable pattern which may be more or less characteristic; but, in the more acute infections, especially those of the respiratory tract, the course of events is so rapid that characteristic patterns do not occur.

The information in the literature concerning the reactions of cells of the respiratory tract to virus infection is limited, but that which is available is rather satisfactory. It is most satisfactory in the case of the influenza, psittacosis, psittacosis-like, and mouse-pneumonitis groups of viruses; and because of the limited time at our disposal,

CELLS OF THE RESPIRATORY TRACT

discussion will be limited to the cellular reactions to those four groups of agents.

INFLUENZA VIRUS INFECTIONS

Specific knowledge of influenza virus infections began with studies by Shope, of swine influenza. Subsequent investigations revealed a strikingly close antigenic relationship between the agents of swine influenza and interpandemic influenza of man. For that and other reasons which cannot be discussed at this time, the swine viruses should be considered strains of influenza virus, and, accordingly, in the present discussion swine influenza will be considered an integral part of the general influenza pattern. The following summary of the cellular reaction in swine influenza is from Shope's Harvey Lecture (2).

Swine influenza. The trachea appears to be little involved. The small bronchi and bronchioles are filled with a polymorphonuclear leucocytic exudate. The cilia of the smaller bronchi are damaged or completely destroyed, and the cytoplasm vacuolated; in places the epithelium is desquamated.

Some alveoli are collapsed and contain desquamated epithelial cells, mononuclear cells, and occasionally coagulated plasma. Leucocytes and red cells are not numerous in the alveoli, although they are almost invariably present. Leucocytes are most abundant in the alveoli which open directly into the terminal bronchioles. The alveolar walls are thickened and infiltrated with round cells. Dilated capillaries in alveolar walls are packed with erythrocytes.

Filtrate disease. Strictly speaking, swine influenza is a complex disease in which the influenza virus and the *Hemophilus influenzae suis* both are essential to the production of the typical clinical disease. Experimental swine virus influenza is a milder disease than the mixed infection, but the differences in cellular reactions are chiefly in degree. In the virus disease (in which bacteria play no part), Shope (2) found the epithelium of the bronchioles damaged and partly desquamated; there was heavy peribronchial cuffing by round cells, and thickening and infiltration of the alveolar walls by monocytes. In contrast to true swine influenza, the collapsed alveoli were free of cells.

Infection of swine with strains of influenza virus obtained from man. Shope and Francis (3) found that although the lesions are less extensive, the reaction of the cells of the respiratory tract of swine to strains of influenza virus (P R 8) obtained from man is indistinguishable from the reaction to strains obtained from swine. As in the cases of infection with the swine strains of virus, the bronchial epithelium was vacuolated and denuded of cilia; the alveolar walls were thickened and infiltrated with monocytes.

Reaction of the cells of the respiratory tract of man to influenza virus infection. Influenza virus infections in man, during interpandemic periods, are relatively mild, and opportunities for histological studies are not frequent. Most of the pathological reports in the literature are concerned with infections in which bacteria played at least a secondary role; and in those studies an exact evaluation of the reactions to the virus alone is difficult. However, in the series reported by Parker, Jolliffe, Barnes, and Finland (4) there were two cases in which the pulmonary lesions clearly seemed to be caused by influenza A virus unassociated with bacteria. Those two cases were especially interesting in that one individual died of heart failure and the other of the pneumonia; it was thus possible to gain information concerning the milder and the more severe reactions.

Parker, Jolliffe, Barnes, and Finland found that necrotizing lesions of bronchi and bronchioles (frequently reported in influenza pneumonias) did not occur in their uncomplicated cases of influenza virus pneumonia; and that in cases complicated by bacterial infection, the necrotic lesions occurred only in the bronchioles in which bacterial invasion was demonstrable.

In the case in which death resulted from heart failure (but in which there was also influenza virus pneumonia) the cellular reaction consisted chiefly of perivascular round cell infiltration, edema of the alveolar walls, and infiltration by monocytes. The epithelium of the bronchioles was unaffected, but the bronchiolar walls were infiltrated with a few lymphocytes, plasma cells, and occasional polymorphonuclear leucocytes. There was swelling of the cells lining the alveoli.

In the second case of uncomplicated pneumonia, death seemed to have been caused directly by the virus pneumonia. The pulmonary lesions differed from those of the milder case, in that the reaction was more intense, but chiefly in that the dilated alveolar ducts and alveoli were lined with dense acidophilic hyaline membranes. Desquamation of epithelium was limited to the alveoli.

Pandemic influenza in man. The hyaline membrane reported by Parker, Jolliffe, Barnes, and Finland is of considerable interest and, perhaps, of importance. It resembles closely the membranes which were observed in cases resulting in death during the 1918 pandemic, and which Goodpasture (5) showed to result from infection by an agent of nonbacterial nature. Goodpasture's description of two cases in which bacteria were not found is as follows:

"The pulmonary lesion to which I would especially refer is a dilated condition of alveolar ducts, with a hyaline membrane partially or completely covering their walls and sometimes those of subtended alveoli . . . The membrane . . . is present most conspicuously in acute pneumonia of short duration. . . . Associated with this lesion are evidences of injury and acute reaction, such as hemorrhage, edema, cellular and fluid exudate and focal necrosis of alveolar walls, . . . This lesion is not to be considered specific in the sense that it contains specific elements in its composition, for so far as has been demonstrated it represents a reaction to injury by elements normally participating in inflammatory processes. The evidence for its specificity depends solely upon the constancy of its association with influenza and its absence in other types of pulmonary inflammation known to be of a different nature. So far as I am aware it has not been described in any inflammation of the lungs other than that accompanying influenza. . . . Two explanations for its presence occur to me. First, that it represents an inflammatory reaction which under circumstances of lowered resistance, such as occur with influenza, may be brought about by any pathogenic microorganism or toxic agent that may gain entrance to the lungs.

"The second explanation is that it represents an inflammatory reaction to an unknown causative agent of influenza which injuries the walls of alveolar ducts at first in a relatively mild degree, causing desquamation and necrosis of epithelial cells and an exudate of large mononuclear cells with some fibrin and serous fluid, all of which become partially concentrated by the inflowing and outflowing respiratory currents of air until they coalesce and adhere to the injured walls."

The similarities of the nonbacterial pneumonias of Goodpasture and the influenza virus pneumonias of Parker, Jolliffe, Barnes, and Finland are striking.

Reaction of the cells of the upper respiratory tract to influenza virus infection. Experimental evidence of the effect of influenza virus on the cells of the upper respiratory tract was furnished by Francis and Stuart-Harris (6), who showed that in ferrets infected by large intranasal doses of influenza A virus there was rapid destruction of the nasal respiratory epithelium. The cellular destruction, organization, and repair were quite nonspecific in that they were indistinguishable from reactions caused by chemical agents.

THE PSITTACOSIS GROUP OF INFECTIONS

In many respects the reaction of the lung to infection by psittacosis virus resembles the reaction to infection by the influenza virus. There are, however, certain rather definite differences which may or may not be of diagnostic significance. In psittacosis the infection appears to begin in the region near the hilum and to spread to adjacent tissue. As a result, it is usually possible to find in the same section various stages of the process.

Psittacosis in monkeys. The following summary is taken from the studies by Rivers and Berry (7) of the experimental disease in monkeys.

Consolidation appears first around the vessels and bronchi near the hilum. In early lesions the alveoli are thickened and edematous and contain leucocytes. The alveolar walls in places are engorged with blood and show some polymorphonuclear or mononuclear infiltration. There is some desquamation of the epithelium. In the definitely consolidated areas, alveolar spaces are filled with leucocytes, chiefly polymorphonuclear. By the fourth day after inoculation the cellular exudate is increased and the alveolar walls more thickened. In some areas near the hilum the alveolar walls are necrotic and the alveolar spaces filled with polymorphonuclear leucocytes and large mononuclear cells. By the sixth day after inoculation giant cells are making their appearance in the alveolar walls, and some mitotic figures are present. As the monkeys improve clinically, the areas of consolidation show organization without connective tissue; and resolution is beginning near the hilum.

Rivers and Berry were unable to find "elementary bodies" in the lungs of their monkeys.

Psittacosis in man. The pulmonary lesions in man are so similar to those observed by Rivers and Berry in monkeys that a detailed description seems unnecessary.

Meningopneumonitis. In 1938, Francis and Magill (8) recovered a virus during their studies of an outbreak of influenza, which in certain respects resembles psittacosis virus; because of the difficulties encountered in obtaining satisfactory serological tests they were unable to determine conclusively whether the virus was obtained from man or whether it originated in the ferrets used in their tests. Subsequently, the same or similar viruses were recovered by several groups of workers from autopsy material after deaths from nonbacterial pneumonias. The following description of the reaction of cells of the lung to infection by the virus of meningopneumonitis is from the case reported by deGara and Furth (9).

The consolidation was predominantly alveolar. In some areas there was interstitial and alveolar edema, with only a few inflammatory cells, while in other places there was massive consolidation characterized by many monocytes and variable numbers of erythrocytes. In the exudate, lymphocytes and monocytes predominated. Many cells of the alveolar lining were desquamated. The authors were of the opinion that the number of epithelial cells free in the alveoli was much greater than was to be expected from desquamation alone, and it seemed to them likely that proliferation had occurred.

There was an eosinophilic hyaline membrane lining many alveoli in areas in which edema fluid was abundant. The mucosa of the bronchi was swollen and in some places the epithelium desquamated; the submucosa was edematous and infiltrated with many lymphocytes and occasional erythrocytes; small collections of round cells were present around the blood vessels.

In imprints stained with Giemsa the predominant cells were lymphocytes, monocytes, and epithelial cells. Most of the large mononuclear cells were vacuolated and free from inclusion bodies. Several of the large mononuclear cells contained many minute palely stained "coccoid" bodies.

Experimental pneumonia in mice. The cellular reaction following intranasal inoculation in mice with the strain of virus isolated by deGara and Furth was similar to that reported by Francis and Magill (8). But, in addition, deGara and Furth reported that in many of the alveoli of mice which died between the second and fourth days there was a pink-staining homogeneous material, and that elementary bodies were seen in both monocytes and polymorphonuclear leucocytes. The elementary bodies were spherical and tended to occur in small clumps.

MOUSE PNEUMONITIS VIRUSES

Granular bodies characteristic of certain nonbacterial pneumonias in mice. Furth and deGara (10) in 1944 reported pneumonia in mice transmissible in serial passage and characterized by hitherto undescribed "granular bodies." The original group of mice in their serial passage had been inoculated with throat washings obtained from patients with "atypical pneumonia," but the etiological relationship of the agent and the disease in man is uncertain. Furth and deGara found similar granular bodies in the pneumonias produced by the mouse pneumonitis virus of Nigg, but not in the pneumonias produced by the PVM virus of Horsfall and Hahn, nor in those produced by the meningopneumonitis virus. It is of practical interest that they found the granular bodies too fragile to be detected in imprints.

The granular bodies are spherical or oval, and measure approximately 12 to 30 micra in greatest diameter; their shape is sharply defined by a thin capsule or membrane, within which are large numbers of spherical elementary bodies of more or less uniform size. They stain well with Giemsa. Their origin is not clear, but the impression of Furth and deGara is that they may be derived from mononuclear elements.

SUMMARY

The histologically recognizable reactions of cells of the respiratory tract to virus infection seem to be more or less alike when infection is by a virus of the influenza, psittacosis, psittacosis-like, and mouse pneumonitis groups; the chief reaction is one of injury to the epithelium or (if it is not permissible to speak of the epithelium of alveoli) of the lining cells; recognizable degrees of injury are loss of cilia, swelling, vacuolization, and desquamation. There is a suggestion that infection by the meningopneumonitis virus may evoke proliferation of the desquamated epithelium. Edema and thickening of the alveolar walls is a common reaction, but even in the pneumonias in which consolidation is complete, the general alveolar structure remains intact.

Inclusion bodies have not been demonstrated in cells of the respiratory tract in infections by the group of viruses considered. The granular bodies described by Furth and deGara are, perhaps, the most characteristic formations evoked by the viruses considered in the present discussion. However, even these granular bodies appear to be nonspecific in that there is at least a suggestion that they are derived from mononuclear elements in which the virus particles have multiplied.

The inflammatory reaction to infection by the groups included in the discussion also is nonspecific. The inflammatory cells are chiefly monocytes, but polymorphonuclear leucocytes play a role, especially in the early stages of the infection; in the psittacosis-like group of pneumonias, Furth and deGara associate the presence of the polymorphonuclear leucocytes with the presence of the virus particles.

Organization differs somewhat in the different infections considered, but the differences seem to be ones of degree. It seems clear that even the hyaline membrane, commonly associated with fatal influenza virus pneumonias in man, occurs also in infections by the psittacosis-like group of agents. Perhaps, psittacosis pneumonia can be distinguished from pneumonias caused by the other viruses in that in the same lung or even in the same section, various stages of the infectious processes may be observed.

The processes of repair are equally nonspecific. That point is particularly striking in the experiments of Francis and Stuart-Harris (6), in which damage and repair following chemical injury were closely similar to the reactions following influenza virus infection.

REFERENCES

1. Rivers, T. M., *Viral and Rickettsial Infections of Man* (Philadelphia, 1948).
2. Shope, R. E., *The Harvey Lectures*, 1935–36, p. 183 (Baltimore, 1936).
3. Shope, R. E., and T. Francis, Jr., The Susceptibility of Swine to the Virus of Human Influenza, *J. Exp. Med.*, 1936, 64:791.
4. Parker, F., Jr., L. S. Jolliffe, M. W. Barnes, and M. Finland, Pathologic

findings in the lungs of five cases from which influenza virus was isolated, *Am. J. Path.*, 1946, 22:797.
5. Goodpasture, E. W., The significance of certain pulmonary lesions in relation to the etiology of influenza, *Am. J. Med. Sc.*, 1919, 158:863.
6. Francis, T., Jr., and C. H. Stuart-Harris, Studies on the nasal histology of epidemic influenza virus infection in the ferret, *J. Exp. Med.*, 1938, 68:789.
7. Rivers, T. M., and G. P. Berry, Psittacosis. IV, Experimentally induced infections in monkeys, *J. Exp. Med.*, 1931, 54:129.
8. Francis, T., Jr., and T. P. Magill, An unidentified virus producing acute meningitis and pneumonitis in experimental animals, *J. Exp. Med.*, 1938, 68:147.
9. deGara, P. F., and J. Furth, Pneumonia produced by a meningopneumotropic virus, *Arch. Path.*, 1948, 45:474.
10. Furth, J., and P. F. deGara, A granular body characteristic of certain nonbacterial pneumonias of mice, *Proc. Soc. Exp. Biol. & Med.*, 1944, 56:107.

Chapter 12

PROLIFERATIVE LESIONS CAUSED BY VIRUSES AND VIRUS-LIKE AGENTS

By JOHN G. KIDD, *Department of Pathology, The New York Hospital—Cornell Medical Center*

Most of the disease-producing viruses that we now know about bring sickness and death to their cellular hosts, and they do this abruptly as a rule, though sometimes inducing more or less transitory hyperplasia beforehand. A few viruses, by contrast, form a kind of partnership with the cells they infect, parasitic virus and infected host cell proliferating together for shorter or longer periods, and sometimes enduringly. One of the first to perceive this was Borrel (1), who noted in 1903 the hyperplasia brought about initially by smallpox and molluscum contagiosum viruses. Subsequently Philibert (2), Rivers (3), and Shope (4), amongst others, have observed the proliferation induced in cells by numerous viruses, notably those responsible for fowl pox, sheep pox, myxomatosis, fibromatosis, and papillomatosis. Thus the principle is now well founded that viruses can make cells grow as well as cause their death. Some of the facts and implications of this theme will here concern us briefly.

TRANSITORY PROLIFERATION INDUCED IN CELLS BY LETHAL VIRUSES

It is relatively easy to group together a number of virus diseases in which proliferation of the infected cells is followed sooner or later by their necrosis. Such is the sequence of events in fowl pox, which used to be called epithelioma contagiosum because it is at once hyperplastic in character and manifestly infectious (5). So too in sheep pox, molluscum contagiosum, and the fibro-mamyxoma spectrum of lesions (Figs. 1 and 2), necrosis eventually follows proliferation of the infected cells (6); and the same is true in more rapid sequence in variola, vaccinia, herpes, and certain other viral infections (7).

The virus-infected cells are eventually absorbed or cast away in

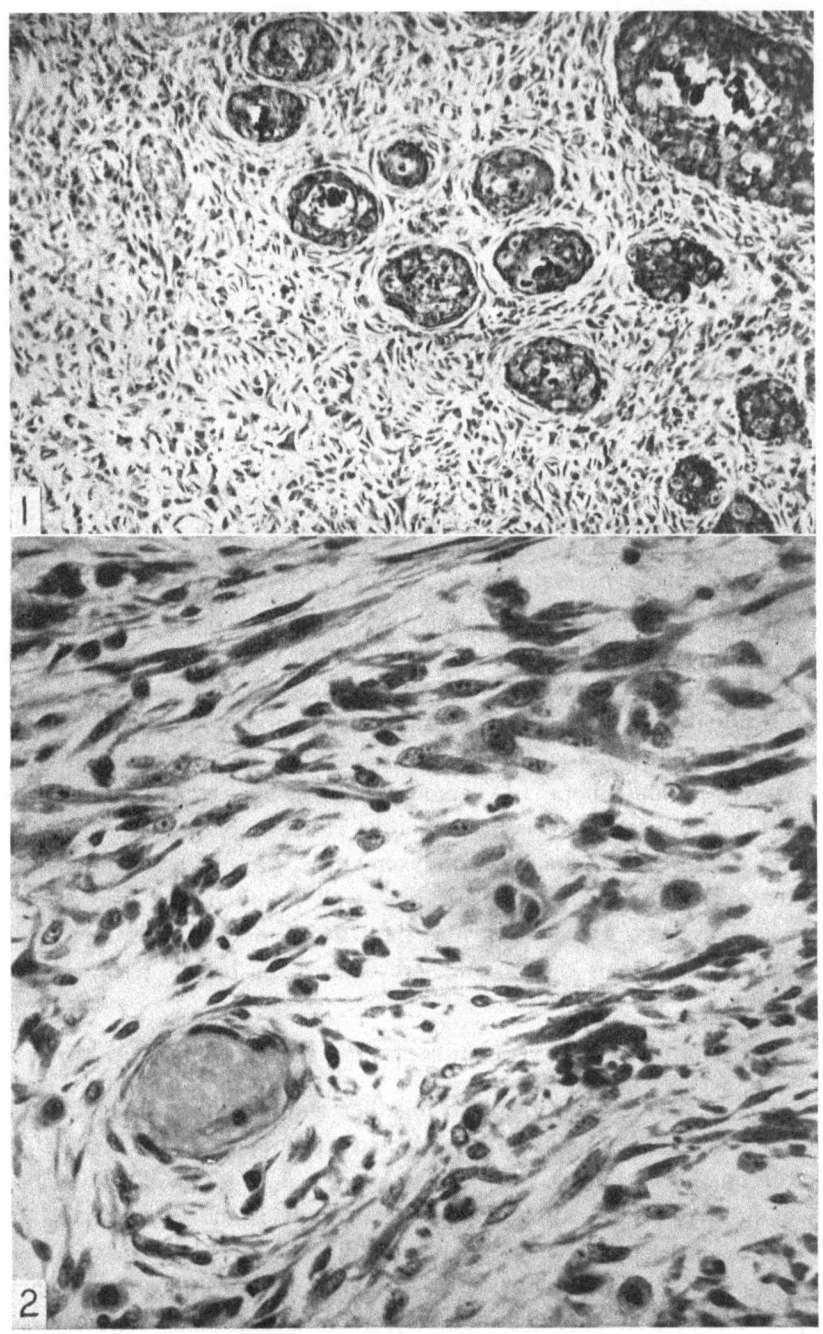

FIGURES 1, 2. THE VIRUS-INDUCED SHOPE FIBROMA IN COTTONTAIL AND IN DOMESTIC RABBITS, RESPECTIVELY (PROVIDED BY DR. SHOPE) Proliferating fibroblasts and islands of epidermal cells that are vacuolated and contain inclusion bodies comprise the lesion. Eventually the fibroblasts die as a result of the virus action, and the lesion regresses, though the course of these events is greatly modified in tarred rabbits (Ahlstrom[6]).

the disease processes just mentioned, and the lesions heal when the viruses are prevented, by the development of neutralizing antibodies or in other ways, from spreading to new cell-hosts. Hence it would seem that virus-induced lesions of this sort differ significantly from the true neoplasms, which are characterized in part by the enduring proliferation of their cells. A number of lesions can be cited, however, in which viruses cause lasting hyperplasia, and their relationship to the tumors seems closer.

ENDURING PROLIFERATION INDUCED IN CELLS BY VIRUSES: THE "CARCINOGENIC" EFFECT OF THE RABBIT PAPILLOMA VIRUS (SHOPE)

It has long been known that viruses cause a variety of papillomata in animals, and several observations indicate that filtrable agents are likewise responsible for certain verrucae in man (8). Perhaps the most extensively studied of the proliferative lesions caused by viruses is the rabbit papillomatosis originally described by Shope (9). Since it may serve as a prototype of lesions of this sort, and since it provides an enlightening example of the relationships that may exist between a virus on the one hand and benign and malignant neoplasia on the other, we may profitably review here certain points in our knowledge of this interesting disease process.

When the Shope virus is rubbed into the scarified skin of normal domestic rabbits it promptly induces a marked proliferation of the epidermal cells (Fig. 3). The germinal cells form into two contiguous layers: a well-defined basal layer composed of a single row of columnar cells, which are arranged in palisade fashion perpendicular to the corium; and outside this a thick layer of differentiating cells which comprise a broad stratum spinosum. The cells of the latter exhibit a distinctive perinuclear vacuolation and dyskeratosis, but they form an orderly mosaic pattern and up to a point mature as do the cells of normal rabbit skin when these undergo hyperplasia for any of a variety of reasons. They do not form characteristic granular and horny layers, however, but instead undergo an atypical cornification, in which a rind of keratin forms about each differentiating cell and fuses with that of its neighbors into a structure like a honeycomb, from which the cell remnants soon disappear. The abnormal keratin adheres firmly, and gradually builds up by accretion from the

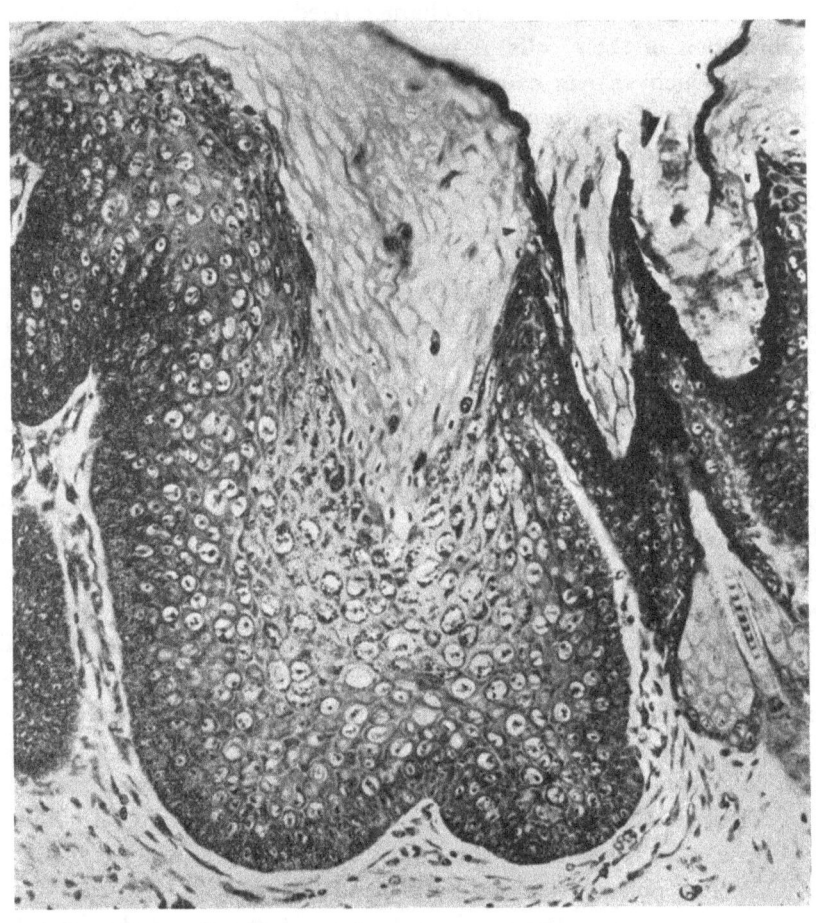

FIGURE 3. BENIGN RABBIT PAPILLOMA INDUCED WITH THE SHOPE VIRUS
Magnification = × 220.

spinosum below into a dry, horny mass that slowly rises one to three centimeters or more above the level of the skin and presently constitutes the bulk of the benign papilloma.

In spite of the abnormalities just mentioned, the papillomas usually remain benign for periods of four to sixteen months or longer. Their basal cells during this time maintain normal polarity and remain sharply separated from the dermis below by a thin basement membrane, which can be impregnated with silver and hence would seem to be composed of reticulin rather than collagen. The cells of the stratum spinosum meanwhile continue to lie in close and orderly apposition to one another, like the tesserae of a compact mosaic, and they likewise continue to differentiate from within outward in orderly sequences as before, displaying conspicuous perinuclear vacuolation and dyskeratosis before they undergo abnormal cornification (Fig. 4). Then more or less abruptly a profound change takes place in the growths, all of those on a given host usually manifesting it within a few weeks' time. When this happens in diagrammatic fashion, the germinal cells, usually in foci near the centers of the papillomas, instead of fitting compactly together into an orderly syncytium as previously, now detach themselves and stand in more or less haphazard relationship to one another, like the elements of an infantry column that had just broken ranks and were about to set out on individual pursuits (Fig. 5). They no longer mature in orderly sequence as they proceed outward from the basal layer, but now take on a new and more or less rigid cellular form. The new cells are much alike and resemble to some extent those formerly composing the lowermost layers of the stratum spinosum; but they differ notably from them in being largely devoid of perinuclear vacuoles and abnormal keratohyalin granules, and in manifesting little or no tendency to undergo abnormal cornification, while showing other differences in nuclear detail and now exhibiting not infrequently abnormal mitoses and degenerating into strange giant forms, especially where poorly nourished. In due course the altered cells replace those of the basal and spinous layers at the focus in which they originated, and they undermine the horny material above it, which sloughs away, exposing raw bleeding tissue underneath; later the changed cells break through the basement membrane and invade the dermis and the panniculus carnosus; eventually they metastasize, and they may

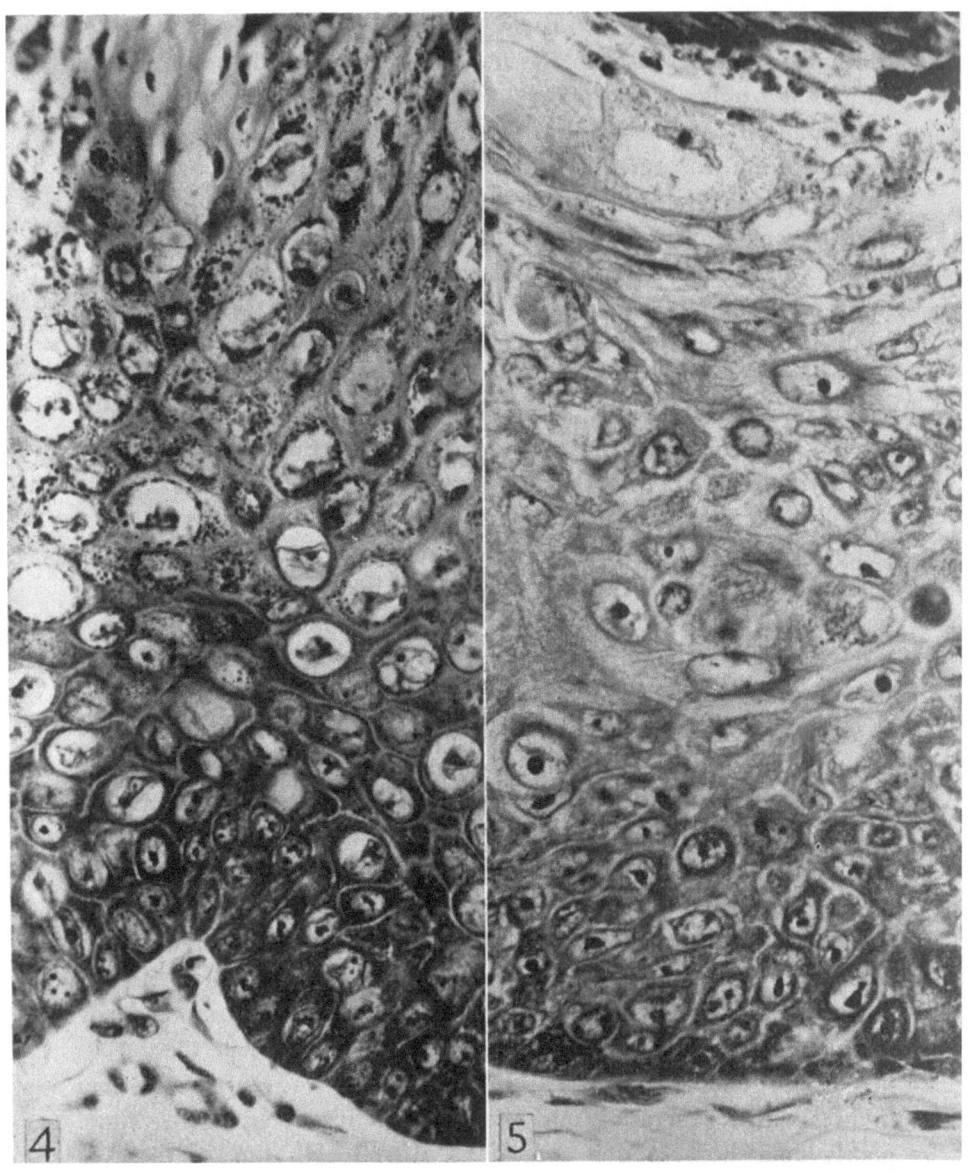

FIGURES 4, 5. THE CELLS OF THE BENIGN PAPILLOMA (FIG. 4) AND THOSE OF A CARCINOMA WHICH RECENTLY ORIGINATED IN ONE OF THE PAPILLOMAS (FIG. 5)
Magnification = × approximately 650.

grow when transplanted to new hosts (10). In sum, the cells of the benign papilloma have become cancerous (11).

The Shope virus obviously causes the orderly proliferation of epidermal cells that comprises the benign rabbit papillomas; but whether it is responsible for their malignant transformation, which comes later, is another matter. The question was complicated at the outset by a curious phenomenon. For while readily recoverable by ordinary means from the benign papillomas which it causes in its natural host (the wild cottontail rabbit), the Shope virus is "masked" in the growths produced with it in domestic rabbits. That is to say, the virus cannot as a rule be extracted from the experimental growths of domestic rabbits, at least not in quantities sufficient to be detectable by the methods ordinarily used (12), and many experiments failed to demonstrate it directly in the cancers (13). Serological and immunological tests have made it plain, however, that the virus is present in the papilloma cells of domestic rabbits, and that it increases in amount as the cells proliferate; for an antibody directed specifically against the virus and detectable by means of neutralization and complement-fixation tests appears in the blood of domestic rabbits carrying the benign growths, or injected with extracts of them, and it increases in titer as the growths enlarge (14). Serological tests of these kinds were applied several years ago to the blood of rabbits that carried one or the other of two transplantable squamous cell cancers that had originated in benign papillomas. When the transplanted cancers had grown progressively, their hosts without exception manifested antibodies that were specific for the papilloma virus (10, 15). Hence it seemed plain that the virus is present in the cancer cells, as well as in the papilloma cells, and reasons were marshaled for supposing that it was the cause of their malignancy (16).

Quite recently, however, a fact has emerged which throws new light on the relationship between the virus and the cancer cells. Mention was just made of the fact that two carcinomas, which had originated in virus-induced papillomas of domestic rabbits, were successfully transplanted several years ago. One of these growths was lost after the second serial transfer, but the second—the V2 carcinoma—has now been transplanted during about twelve years through some sixty tumor generations. Much evidence indicates that the papilloma virus persisted in the cells of the V2 carcinoma during the first five years

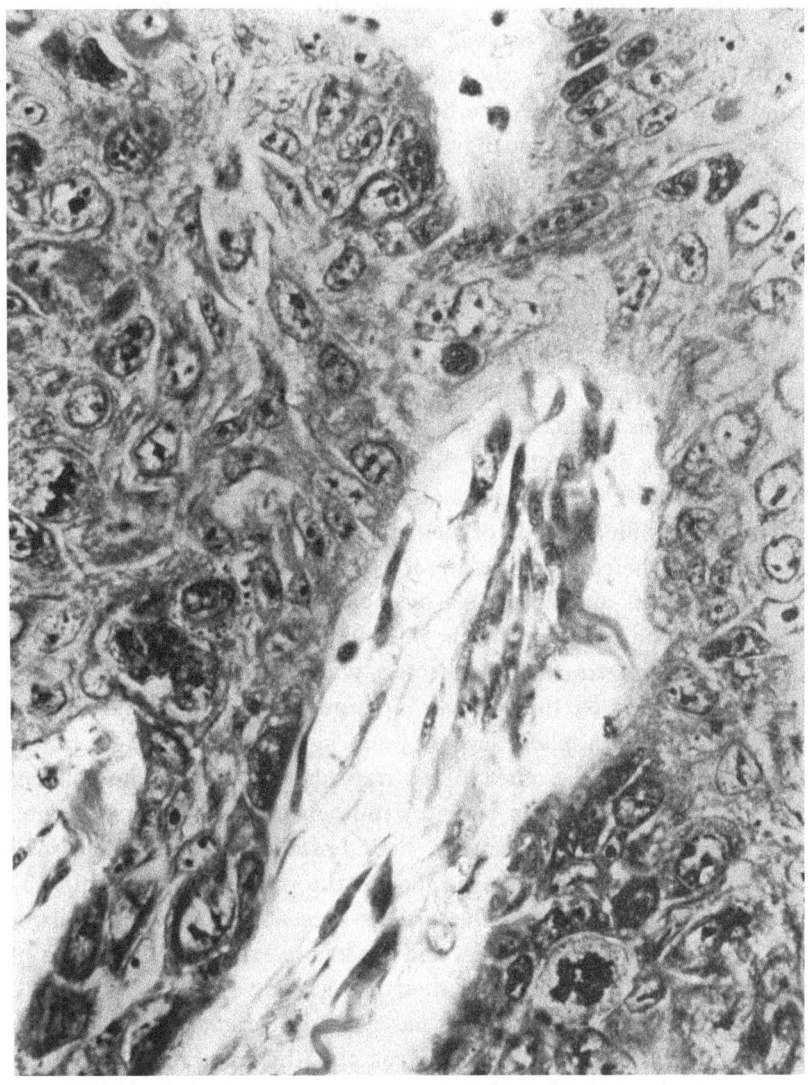

FIGURE 6. A CARCINOMA THAT HAS NOW INVADED THE DERMIS AND EXTENDED LATERALLY BENEATH A VIRUS-INDUCED PAPILLOMA FROM WHICH IT RECENTLY ORIGINATED

The cells of all such growths tested thus far have contained the Shope papilloma virus in masked or altered form (10, 15, 17). Compare with Fig. 7. Magnification = × 700.

following their initial transplantation; for every one of more than 100 animals in which the cancer grew progressively in the twenty-two tumor generations transplanted during this time provided blood that contained the specific antibody for the papilloma virus (10, 15).

Since the association between the virus and the cancer cells appeared to be quite stable, it seemed reasonable to discontinue the serological tests during the war as a means of conservation. When they were resumed at its end, the antibody for the papilloma virus was not present in the blood of rabbits that had long carried progressively enlarging V2 carcinomas of the forty-sixth tumor generation (about ten years after the initial transplantation); the same has been true in all tests made thus far with blood from animals carrying tumors of subsequent generations (17). Manifestly the antigenic papilloma virus disappeared from the V2 carcinoma cells sometime between the twenty-second and forty-sixth tumor generations. Whether it played a significant part in the intracellular activities of the V2 carcinoma cells during the first twenty-two serial transfers, or whether it merely rode along as a passenger—as extraneous viruses sometimes do in transplanted cancer cells (18 and 19)—only to be crowded out later, perhaps by some more essential cellular constituent, is of course problematical (20, 21). But it seems clear that the papilloma virus per se is not essential for the continuing malignancy of the V2 carcinoma cells; for these are now, in the absence of the virus, no less malignant than they were when they carried it, and they do not differ notably otherwise, if one may judge from morphological and biological criteria (Figs. 6, 7). Hence there is reason for placing the Shope virus, along with tar, arsenic, sunlight, methylcholanthrene, and a host of other substances, in the category of so-called carcinogenic agents—agents, that is to say, which change tissues so that cancers arise in them but which play no essential part in the continuing malignancy of the cancer cells.

PROLIFERATIVE LESIONS CAUSED BY VIRUS-LIKE AGENTS

It is hardly possible to pursue our theme further without running into the problem of what viruses are. This is not the time or place to argue whether they are protein molecules (22), simplified parasites (23, 24), or microbial midgets of diverse sorts (25), much less to

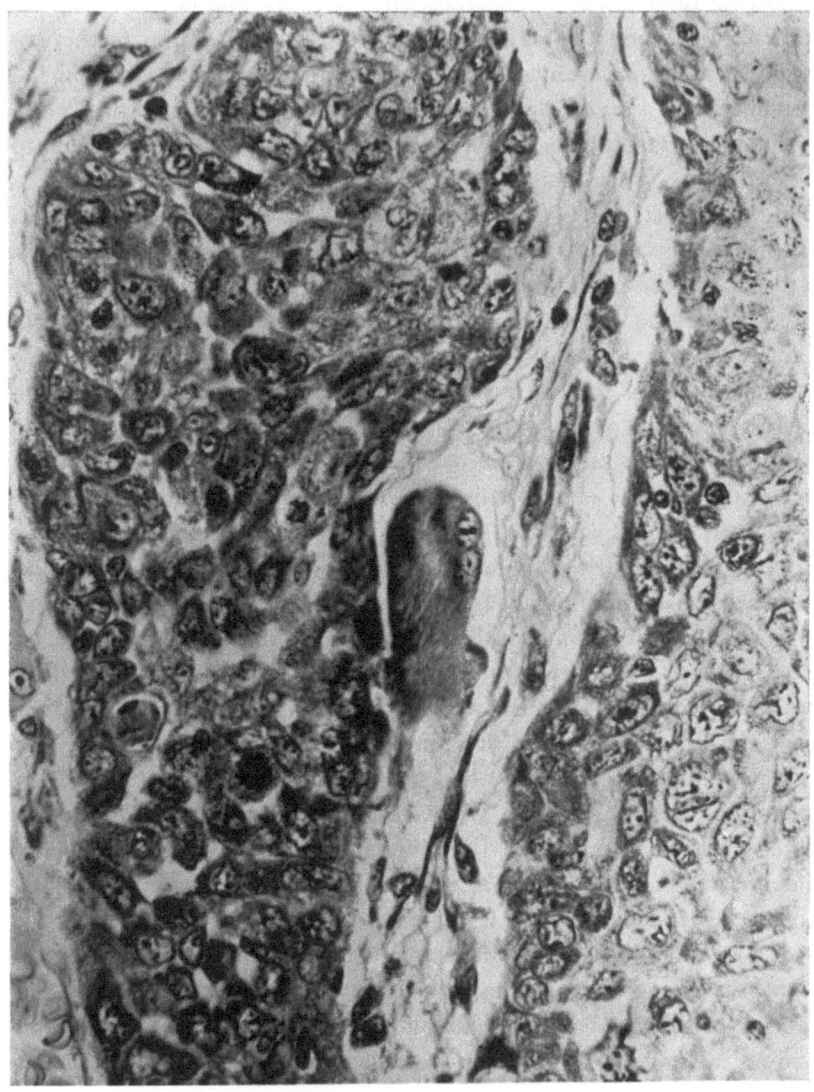

FIGURE 7. THE V₂ CARCINOMA AFTER FIFTY-FOUR SERIAL TRANSPLANTATIONS DURING ABOUT TWELVE YEARS IN NORMAL RABBITS
The papilloma virus disappeared from its cells between the twenty-second and forty-sixth tumor generations (see text) without causing any noteworthy change in their morphological or biological characters. Compare with Fig. 6. Magnification = × 700.

attempt to say whether they evolved initially from things extrinsic or intrinsic to cells of the kinds they now prey upon (26, 27). Even so, it may prove profitable to keep these questions in mind as we review briefly the properties and effects of several filtrable agents that are certainly virus-like, even though their attributes as now known may not suffice, in the view of some, to distinguish them as viruses.

The first amongst the virus-like agents responsible for proliferative lesions are those causing a variety of mesenchymal neoplasms in fowls. Soon after it had been shown that a filtrable agent causes epithelioma contagiosum (fowl pox), Ellerman and Bang (28) learned that other agents of this sort are responsible for various leukoses or leukemias in chickens, and a few years later Rous and his associates (29) found that several distinctive agents can be extracted from as many kinds of sarcomas in chickens, each agent reproducing, under suitable experimental conditions, growths of the type from which it had come (29). These findings have been abundantly confirmed during the past forty years, and extended here and there (30, 31); they constitute the bulk of what is known today about cellular factors that actually cause cancer (20, 21). Yet the point deserves emphasis that the precise nature of the filtrable agents responsible for the fowl sarcomas remains undisclosed, while furthermore next to nothing has been learned about the mode of spread of the filtrable agents from infected to susceptible hosts in nature, and about the ways they produce their effects within cells (Fig. 8 [32]).

A second virus-like agent that causes interesting proliferative lesions has more recently come into prominence. This is the so-called milk factor (33, 34), which, with the aid of estrogenic stimulation, causes adenomatous hyperplasia of mammary epithelium in certain strains of mice (35, 36, 37, Fig. 9 [38]). It is plain that the milk factor passes from teat to mouth during suckling and increases in amount as it sojourns in host after host, and furthermore that it shares with the sedimentable constituents of normal tissue cells certain of the physical and chemical properties of viruses. Yet much remains to be learned about its nature and effects. It resembles the constituents of normal tissue cells more than it does the viruses in lacking antigenicity in its native species, while its relationship to the cancers that arise in the proliferating mammary acini of susceptible mice remains wholly conjectural. Indeed it is conceivable that an entirely different cellular factor may be responsible for the change to cancer, and that the milk factor, like the Shope papilloma virus, while "carcinogenic" in the limited sense of causing benign adenomas that later

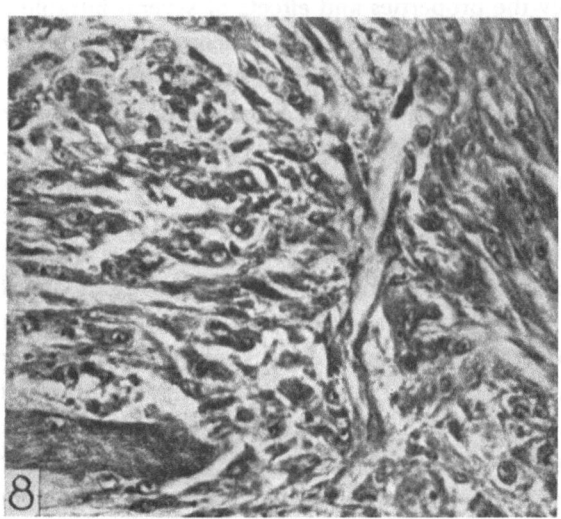

FIGURE 8. CHICKEN TUMOR—10—ONE OF THE SARCOMAS ORIGINALLY FOUND BY ROUS AND MURPHY TO YIELD A FILTRABLE AGENT BY MEANS OF WHICH THE GROWTH CAN BE REPRODUCED IN NORMAL FOWLS

Claude, Porter, and Pickels (32), using the electron microscope, have recently found "colonies" of spherical bodies in the cytoplasm of the cells of this sarcoma which they feel represent its causative agent.

become malignant, may turn out to be an epiphenomenon so far as the continuing causation of malignancy is concerned.

A third virus or virus-like agent probably responsible for proliferative effects in tissue cells has been studied by Lucké who found that certain renal carcinomas in frogs are made up of cells often containing conspicuous acidophilic intranuclear inclusion bodies, and that they yield a filtrable agent which withstands desiccation and glycerination and by means of which the growths can be reproduced experimentally, though this is accomplished only sporadically and after a long incubation period (39). The properties of the filtrable agent have not yet been completely studied, and no proof exists that it is the continuing cause of malignancy in the cells it inhabits.

A fourth virus-like agent that is regularly associated with proliferating cells was described in 1938, when the fact was recorded that a distinctive substance having certain properties remarkably similar to those of the viruses can be identified by serological means

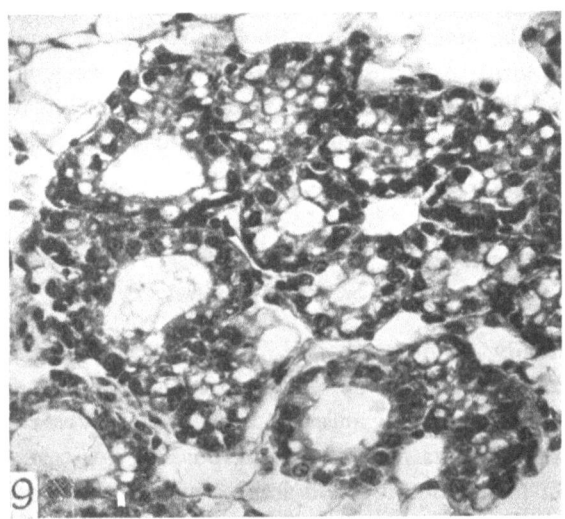

FIGURE 9. ONE OF NUMEROUS HYPERPLASTIC NODULES IN THE MAMMARY GLANDS OF A DBA FEMALE BREEDER MOUSE (PROVIDED BY DR. KIRSHBAUM)

It illustrates the hyperplasia of mammary acini that presumably results from the combined action of estrogenic hormones and the viruslike milk factor. Hyperplastic nodules of this sort are often numerous in the mammary growths of old female mice that carry the milk factor, and some of them seem to give rise to malignant adenocarcinomas, though the precise relationship of the milk factor to the cancers remains to be determined. By means of electron microscopy Porter and Thompson (38) have recently disclosed particulate bodies associated with epithelial cells from mammary cancers of mice carrying the milk factor.

in extracts of the Brown-Pearce carcinoma of rabbits (40). Many facts showed plainly that the virus-like material can be extracted regularly and in large amounts from the Brown-Pearce carcinoma cells, but no trace of it could be found in extracts of other rabbit tissues, either normal or neoplastic. When tested in various ways, however, the distinctive substance did not manifest the ability to induce neoplasia or other changes in a variety of rabbit tissue cells, so that it could not be classified as a virus. Furthermore, for some time evidence was not at hand to indicate whether it has anything to do with the proliferative activities of the carcinoma cells with which it is naturally associated. Recently, however, the fact has been recorded that the growth of living Brown-Pearce carcinoma cells is suppressed by the action of the antibody that reacts specifically with its distinctive virus-like constituent[1] (21, 41). Hence it appears possible that the distinctive substance may be responsible for the proliferation of the carcinoma cells, though this does not necessarily follow.

PROLIFERATIVE LESIONS OF UNKNOWN CAUSE, POSSIBLY INDUCED BY VIRUSES OR VIRUS-LIKE AGENTS

As has already been mentioned, viruses or virus-like agents are known to cause several of the benign papillomata and at least one type of benign adenoma in animals, and scattered observations indicate that similar agents may also be responsible for several kinds of papillomas in man, notably condyloma acuminatum, common warts, and possibly also certain laryngeal papillomas (8, 42). It is furthermore commonly supposed that agents of this sort may also be responsible for intraductal papillomas of the breast and papillomas of the urinary bladder in human beings, growths of both types being often multiple in a given host and not infrequently undergoing malignant transformation. Other proliferative lesions of man and animals could readily be listed which are possibly caused by filtrable pathogens; as in the examples already cited, however, little or no evidence exists to support the supposition that filtrable viruses are actually responsible for them.

There is perhaps more reason for supposing that a filtrable agent may be responsible for a relatively uncommon neoplasm of human beings which is variously called pulmonary adenomatosis and "alveolar cell" carcinomatosis. The gross and microscopic characters of this neoplastic disease distinguish it sharply from the usual primary and secondary cancers of the lung in man, though the lesion seems practically identical with that seen in Jaagsiekte, an infectious disease of

---

[1] Burmester more recently still (*Cancer Research*, 1947, 7:459–467) has noted similar effects produced by an antibody against the cells of an avian lymphoid tumor.

sheep which is probably virus-induced (43, 44). Yet here again proof is lacking that the disease in man is infectious or that it is caused by a filtrable agent (45, 46).

To illustrate certain of the difficulties inherent in experimentation designed to test for causative viruses in proliferative lesions of unknown cause, several facts now at hand should perhaps be listed seriatim. Firstly, the best studied of the growth-producing viruses—those causing papillomas in man and animals—have remarkably restricted cellular affinities, some attacking epidermis but not other epithelium (8, 47), while others produce papillomas only in the oral mucosa (48). Secondly, none of the viruses or virus-like agents responsible for neoplastic proliferation in mammals has thus far been propagated in chick-embryo cells, and few or none have proved pathogenic in species of animals distant from that in which they naturally occur. Thirdly, the papillomas elicited by tarring the skin of rabbits, while exhibiting a number of histological and biological features in common with growths caused by the Shope virus, regularly failed in a number of experiments to yield a causative agent (49). Certain implications of these facts will be mentioned further on.

SUMMARY AND COMMENT

In this brief review the observation has been recalled that viruses can make cells grow, as well as cause their death. A distinction has been made, however, between those viral diseases, exemplified by fowl pox, sheep pox, molluscum contagiosum, and the fibroma-myxoma spectrum, in which proliferation is followed by necrosis of the virus-infected cells, and the true tumors, in which enduring cellular proliferation largely characterizes the lesion. A variety of papillomata were cited as examples of lesions in which viruses cause persisting hyperplasia, but no attempt was made to say whether these lesions should be classified as tumors.

In the most extensively studied of the proliferative lesions due to actual viruses—that induced in rabbits by the Shope papilloma virus—it was pointed out that the virus is "carcinogenic," in the sense that the benign papilloma cells, proliferating as result of its action, eventually undergo malignant transformation. The virus cannot be held responsible for the continuing malignancy of the transformed cells, however, for serological tests indicate that it eventually disappeared from them when they were held long under observation, though their malignancy was not lessened and their proliferative vigor remained undiminished when the virus disappeared.

Since all is not yet certain about the origin, nature, and effects of viruses, it seemed reasonable to consider in this review the effects of several filtrable agents that have been isolated from proliferative lesions but whose properties as defined thus far hardly suffice to distinguish them as viruses. Amongst these agents, herein termed virus-like, are the following: those responsible for a variety of leukoses and sarcomas in fowls; the so-called milk factor, which, in concert with estrogenic hormones, causes adenomatous hyperplasia of mammary acini in mice; the filtrable agent implicated in renal carcinomatosis of leopard frogs; and the distinctive virus-like constituent which is regularly associated with Brown-Pearce carcinoma cells of rabbits, and which may be responsible for their proliferation. Brief mention was made of the uncertainties now existing about the nature of these virus-like agents and about their effects on cells.

In addition a number of proliferative lesions of unknown cause, possibly induced by viruses or virus-like agents, were cited, and certain of the difficulties now inherent in experimentation designed to test for causative agents in proliferative lesions were enumerated.

Finally the point deserves mention that the instances in which viruses or virus-like agents have been found in association with proliferative lesions are exceedingly few in number, especially when contrasted with the innumerable examples of growths in man and animals from which no such agents have yet been got. Even so, the viruses and virus-like agents are conspicuous amongst the factors now known to cause abnormal and enduring proliferation in differentiated cells, while furthermore the attempts made thus far to identify such agents in tumors of unknown cause, though numerous and repeated, have in no sense been exhaustive, and they have all had to be made with an understanding of intracellular constituents and intracellular processes at best but rudimentary. To learn more about the viruses and virus-like agents in this relation is a pointed task for modern pathology; its prosecution, one may venture, could well give rise to an intracellular pathology undreamed of by Virchow.

REFERENCES

1. Borrel, A., Epithelioses infectieuses et epitheliomas, *Ann. Inst. Pasteur*, 1903, 17:81.
2. Philibert, A., Virus cytotropes (virus filtrants-virus filtrables), *Ann. de Med.*, 1924, 16:283.
3. Rivers, T. M., Some general aspects of pathological conditions caused by filtrable viruses, *Am. J. Path.*, 1928, 4:91. Infectious myxomatosis of rabbits, observations on the pathological changes induced by virus myxomatosum (Sanarelli), *J. Exp. Med.*, 1930, 51:965.
4. Shope, R. E., A filtrable virus causing a tumor-like condition in rabbits and its relationship to virus myxomatosum, *J. Exp. Med.*, 1932, 56:803.
5. Goodpasture, E. W., Virus diseases of fowls as exemplified by contagious epithelioma (fowl pox) of chickens and pigeons, in *Filtrable Viruses*, pp. 235–270, T. M. Rivers, ed. (Baltimore, 1928).
6. Ahlstrom, C. G., and C. H. Andrewes, Fibroma virus infection in tarred rabbits, *J. Path. & Bact.*, 1938, 47:65.
7. Rivers, T. M., Filtrable viruses with particular reference to psittacosis, The Harvey Lectures, Series XXIX, 1933–34, pp. 220–244.
8. Findlay, G. M., in *A System of Bacteriology in Relation to Medicine*, vol. 7, pp. 252–257, Great Britain, Medical Research Council, (London, His Majesty's Stationery Office, 1930).
9. Shope, R. E., Infectious papillomatosis of rabbits, *J. Exp. Med.*, 1933, 58:607.
10. Kidd, J. G., and P. Rous, A transplantable rabbit carcinoma originating in a virus-induced papilloma and containing the virus in masked or altered form, *J. Exp. Med.*, 1940, 71:813.
11. Rous, P., and J. W. Beard, The progression to carcinoma of virus-induced rabbit papillomas (Shope), *J. Exp. Med.*, 1935, 62:523.
12. Friedewald, W. F., and J. G. Kidd, The recoverability of virus from papillomas produced therewith in domestic rabbits, *J. Exp. Med.*, 1944, 79:591.
13. Kidd, J. G., and P. Rous, Cancers deriving from the virus papillomas of wild rabbits under natural conditions, *J. Exp. Med.*, 1940, 71:469.
14. Kidd, J. G., Antigenicity and infectivity of extracts of virus-induced rabbit papillomas, *Proc. Soc. Exp. Biol. & Med.*, 1938, 37:657. Immunological reactions with a virus causing papillomas in rabbits; I: Demonstration of complement fixation reaction: relation of virus-neutralizing and complement-binding antibodies, II: Properties of the complement binding antigen present in extracts of the growths: Its relation to the virus, III: Antigenicity and pathogenicity of extracts of the growths of wild and domestic species: General discussion, *J. Exp. Med.*, 1938, 68:703. The masking effect of extravasated antibody on the rabbit papilloma virus (Shope), *J. Exp. Med.*, 1939, 70:583. The detection of a "masked" virus (the Shope papilloma virus) by means of immuniza-

tion, results of immunization with mixtures containing virus and antibody, *J. Exp. Med.*, 1941, 74:321.
15. Kidd, J. G., The enduring partnership of neoplastic virus and carcinoma cells, continued increase of virus in the V₂ carcinoma during propagation in virus-immune hosts, *J. Exp. Med.*, 1942, 75:7.
16. Rous, P., The virus tumors and the tumor problem, *Am. J. Cancer*, 1936, 28:233. The nearer causes of cancer, *J.A.M.A.*, 1943, 122:573. Concerning the cancer problem. *Am. Scientist*, 1946, 34:329.
17. Smith, W. E., J. G. Kidd, and P. Rous, Recovery and disappearance of the rabbit papilloma virus (Shope) from the carcinomas that originate from papilloma cells, *Proc. Fourth International Cancer Research Congress*, St. Louis, 1947, p. 84.
18. Levaditi, C., and S. Nicolau, Affinité du virus herpétique pour les néoplasmes épithéliaux, *Compt. rend, soc. de Biol.*, 1922, 87:498.
Levaditi, C., R. Schoen, and L. Reininé. Virus de la peste aviare et tumour de Pearce, *Compt. rend. soc. de Biol.*, 1937, 124:711.
19. Rivers, T. M., and L. Pearce, Growth and persistence of filtrable viruses in a transplantable neoplasm, *J. Exp. Med.*, 1925, 42:523.
20. Kidd, J. G., Viruses and virus-like agents as causes of cancer, a brief recounting and reflection, *Bull. Johns Hopkins Hosp.*, 1948, 82:583.
21. Kidd, J. G., Distinctive constituents of tumor cells and their possible relations to the phenomena of autonomy, anaplasia, and cancer causation, Cold Spring Harbor Symposia on Quantitative Biology: Heredity and variation in microorganisms, Cold Spring Harbor, Long Island Biological Association, 1946, 11:94.
22. Stanley, W. M., The isolation and properties of tobacco mosaic and other virus proteins, The Harvey Lectures, Series XXXIII, 1937–38, pp. 170–204.
23. Green, R. G., On the nature of filtrable viruses, *Science*, 1935, 82:443.
24. Laidlaw, Sir Patrick, *Virus Diseases and Viruses* (The Rede Lecture, Cambridge University Press, England, 1938).
25. Rivers, T. M., The nature of viruses, *Physiol. Rev.*, 1932, 12:423.
26. Dale, Sir Henry, A prospect in therapeutics, *Brit. Med. J.*, 1943, 2:411.
27. Haddow, A., Transformation of cells and viruses, *Nature*, 1944, 154:194.
28. Ellermann, V., and O. Bang, Experimentelle leukemie bei huhnern, *Zbl. Bakt. Orig.*, 1908, 46:595.
Ellermann, V., *The Leucosis of Fowls and Leucemia Problems* (London, 1921).
29. Rous, P., A transmissible avian neoplasm (sarcoma of the common fowl), *J. Exp. Med.*, 1910, 12:696. A sarcoma of the fowl transmissible by an agent separable from the tumor cells, *J. Exp. Med.*, 1911, 23:397.
30. Claude, A., and J. B. Murphy, Transmissible tumors of the fowl, *Physiol. Rev.*, 1933, 13:246.

31. Foulds, L., Filtrable tumors of fowls: A critical review, Supplement to *Eleventh Scientific Report of the Imperial Cancer Research Fund* (London, 1934).
32. Claude, A., K. R. Porter, and E. G. Pickels, Electron microscope study of chicken tumor cells, *Cancer Research*, 1947, 7:421.
33. Bittner, J. J., Some possible effects of nursing on the mammary gland tumor incidence in mice, *Science*, 1936, 84:162. Possible relationships of the estrogenic hormones, genetic susceptibility and milk influence in the production of mammary cancer in mice, *Cancer Research*, 1942, 2:710.
34. Andervont, H. B., The mammary tumor agent and its implications in cancer research, *Yale J. Biol. Med.*, 1946, 18:333.
35. Pullinger, B. D., Forced activation and early detection of the milk-borne agent of mammary adenomas in mice, *Brit. J. Cancer*, 1947, 1:177.
36. Bonser, G. M., A microscopical study of the evolution of mouse mammary cancer, the effect of the milk factor and a comparison with the human disease, *J. Path & Bact.*, 1945, 57:413.
37. Kirschbaum, A., W. L. Williams, and J. J. Bittner, Induction of mammary cancer with methylcholanthrene, I: Histogenesis of the induced neoplasm, *Cancer Research*, 1946, 6:354.
38. Porter, K. R., and H. P. Thompson, A particulate body associated with epithelial cells cultured from mammary carcinomas of mice of a milk-factor strain, *J. Exp. Med.*, 1948, 88:15.
39. Lucké, B., A neoplastic disease of the kidney of the frog, *Rana pipiens*, *Am. J. Cancer*, 1934, 20:352. Carcinoma in the leopard frog, its probable causation by a virus, *J. Exp. Med.*, 1938, 68:457.
40. Kidd, J. G., A complement-binding antigen in extracts of the Brown-Pearce carcinoma of rabbits, *Proc. Soc. Exp. Biol. & Med.*, 1938, 38:292. A distinctive substance associated with the Brown-Pearce rabbit carcinoma, I: Presence and specificity of the substance as determined by serum reactions, II: Properties of the substance, discussion, *J. Exp. Med.*, 1940, 71:335.
    MacKenzie, I., and J. G. Kidd, Incidence and specificity of the antibody for a distinctive constituent of the Brown-Pearce tumor, *J. Exp. Med.*, 1945, 82:41.
41. Kidd, J. G., Supression of growth of the Brown-Pearce tumor by a specific antibody, *Science*, 1944, 99:348. Suppression of growth of Brown-Pearce tumor cells by a specific antibody, with a consideration of the nature of the reacting cell constituent, *J. Exp. Med.* 1946, 83:227.
42. Rivers, T. M., in *Viral and Rickettsial Infections of Man*, pp. 2-5 (Philadelphia), 1948.
43. Bonné, C., Morphological resemblance of pulmonary adenomatosis (jaagsiekte) in sheep and certain cases of cancer of the lung in man, *Amer. J. Cancer*, 1939, 35:491.

44. Dungal, N., Experiments with jaggsiekte, *Am. J. Path.*, 1946, 22:737.
45. Neuberger, K. T., and E. F. Geever, Alveolar cell tumor of the human lung, *Arch. Path.*, 1942, 33:551.
46. Simon, M. A., So-called pulmonary adenomatosis and "alveolar cell tumors," report of a case, *Am. J. Path.*, 1947, 23:413.
47. Kidd, J. G., and R. G. Parsons, Tissue affinity of Shope papilloma virus, *Proc. Soc. Exp. Biol. & Med.*, 1936, 35:438.
48. Parsons, R. J., and J. G. Kidd, Oral papillomatosis of rabbits, a virus disease, *J. Exp. Med.*, 1943, 77:233.
49. Rous, P., and J. G. Kidd, A comparison of virus-induced rabbit tumors with the tumors of unknown cause elicited by tarring, *J. Exp. Med.*, 1939, 69:399.

Chapter 13

THE PATHOLOGY OF LYMPHOCYTIC CHORIOMENINGITIS VIRUS INFECTION: A DISCUSSION

BY R. D. LILLIE, *National Institutes of Health*

WHILE REPORTS of nontuberculous lymphocytic meningitides with usually favorable clinical outcome date back almost to the introduction of spinal fluid examination as a routine diagnostic procedure, it is evident from scanning the literature that many of the cases in this group had other etiologies. Blau's report (1) was of a case of internal hydrocephalus and chronic serous meningitis secondary to a chronic postmeasles, purulent otitis media. Beneke's report (2) was concerned with the chronic posttraumatic fibrocystic meningitides. Rizzo's series (3) comprised cases of aseptic meningitis induced by intrathecal serum injections, both therapeutic in man and experimental in animals.

Until Armstrong (4) isolated the virus from a case in the St. Louis encephalitis outbreak of 1933, the identification of the specific etiologic entity now called lymphocytic choriomeningitis was not possible. It is probable that Margulis's series (5) of fifteen nonfatal cases of lymphocytic and serous meningitides included at least some cases of this entity.

The case from which Armstrong's first strain was isolated was considered to be one of encephalitis due to the St. Louis virus. The brain and cord presented few foci of generally scanty perivascular lymphocyte infiltration in the cerebral cortex, basal ganglia, thalamus, and gray substance of the spinal cord. In the pons there were more numerous vascular infiltrations in which some plasma cells and macrophages were mingled with the predominating lymphocytes. Also, some small glia nodes were noted in the pontile nuclei. The meninges presented slight focal infiltration by lymphocytes, plasma cells, and macrophages. The chorioid plexus of the lateral ventricle was slightly fibrosed, and the anterior horn cells of the spinal cord presented partial tigrolysis and some pigmentation. No midbrain or medulla was included in the available material. Otherwise, a serosanguinopurulent lobular pneumonia was the principal lesion found.

At the time, this case was considered to be one of St. Louis encephalitis and formed part of the material studied by McCordock, Collier, and Gray (6). In view of the paucity and relatively mild character of the encephalitic lesions in this case and of the presence of minor numbers of perivascular lesions and glia nodes in the brains of some monkeys infected with the lymphocytic choriomeningitis virus (7), I have entertained some doubts as to the exact etiologic nature of the process seen.

Armstrong's second strain of virus was recovered from the brain of a woman who died after a three-day illness. There was abrupt onset, with headache, chill, fever of 104.6° F., and delirium. On the next day the neck was stiff, and spinal fluid presented a pleocytosis of 200 cells, chiefly lymphocytes. The second puncture fluid was bloody. The brain lesions comprised necrosing cellular thrombi, focal purulent to karyorrhectic necrosis with many staphylococci, and arteriolar necroses with infarction of surrounding white substance. There were also a few scattered focal glioses of loosely packed slender glia cells and scattered small vessels with endothelial swelling and sheath lymphocyte infiltration. The meninges presented patches of lymphocyte and plasma cell infiltration and of polymorphonuclear and macrophage infiltration.

Again, it remains dubious whether the lesions in this case were assignable primarily to the virus, with secondary purulent encephalitis, or whether the presence of the virus was coincidental.

The virus was also isolated from the brain in both, and from the blood in one and the lung in the other, of the cases of Smadel, Green, Paltauf, and Gonzales (8). They reported perivascular lymphocyte infiltration in the meninges, brain, liver, and other (unspecified) organs of their second case only, as well as a subdural hematoma. An extensive necrotizing pharyngitis was present in one of their cases. Focal pneumonia was present in both cases. In the one with no brain lesions the exudate varied from polymorphonuclear leucocytes to mononuclear cells; in the other there was septal infiltration by mononuclears and an exudate of large mononuclears, red cells, and fibrin.

Howard (9) reported on a series of eight cases from which the virus was isolated from spinal fluid during life or from the brain. Of these cases, three were fatal and autopsies were reported on the last two. Serum protection tests were not mentioned. One of the nonfatal cases presented a slight pleocytosis (15 cells) but no clinical meningeal signs. Another was clinically meningitis. The remaining six were clinically diagnosed as encephalitis, and two of the nonfatal cases gave spinal fluid cell counts of less than five cells per cubic millimeter.

In Howard's case 7 (7 days), Zimmermann described massive areas of necrosis of gray and white substance in the spinal cord, with hemorrhage, and with perivascular and meningeal infiltration chiefly by polymorphonuclears, neuronolysis, and myelinophagia. Outside of necrosing areas, extensive ischemic changes of anterior horn cells were noted. In the brain there were many vascular lesions, especially in the white substance and in the substantia nigra. Endothelial swelling and proliferation, perivascular lymphocyte and plasma cell infiltration, perivenous parenchymal infiltration by polymorphonuclear leucocytes, and, grossly, petechial hemorrhage were noted. There were also numerous paravascular nodules of microglia, astrocytes, and fat granule cells.

In Howard's case 8 (9 days), Zimmermann reported extensive hemorrhagic necrosis of the frontal lobes, more on the right, with replacement by numerous monocytes, leucocytes, and microglia, much capillary endothelial proliferation and occlusion, focal necrosis, and vessel sheath infiltration by plasma cells. The chorioid plexus was not involved, but there was much infiltration of the cerebrospinal meninges by lymphocytes, plasma cells, and large mononuclear cells which often contained prominent "pink-staining" bodies.

In both of Howard's autopsy cases there was also a focal pneumonia, which was not described microscopically. Descriptions of the other viscera were not included.

The paralytic case reported clinically by MacCallum and Findlay (10) was probably similar in general nature. This was a 17-year-old girl who developed persistent paralysis of the lower extremities shortly after the onset of an acute febrile attack. While the case was first diagnosed as poliomyelitis, virus studies revealed the presence of lymphocytic choriomeningitis virus in guinea pigs inoculated with spinal fluid taken on the sixth day, and in a monkey and guinea pigs inoculated later with nasal washings. No tests were made for the presence of antibodies against the virus in the patient's serum.

Findlay, Alcock, and Stern (11) recorded lower-extremity and bladder paralysis which later cleared up in one of their two cases, left-facial and bilateral lower-extremity paralysis in the other. Virus strains were recovered from both.

Riggs's case (12) was the single fatality in the series of thirty-seven cases reported by Noone (13), about which cases Noone says: "Material . . . was not infectious for guinea pigs, mice, rabbits, or monkeys. Further, the convalescent serums afforded no protection against the virus of acute choriomeningitis. Neutralization tests were negative against . . . St. Louis . . . encephalitis" and poliomyelitis of the 1931 Philadelphia and mixed strains

The autopsy case presented perivascular hemorrhage in the walls of the third ventricle; mild perivascular lymphocyte and mast cell infiltration in the white substance; swelling, edema, and ischemic degeneration of nerve cells in the tuber cinereum and medulla, of Purkinje cells in the cerebellum, and of anterior horn cells in the spinal cord; generalized degeneration of capillary endothelia and perivascular edema, and peripheral demyelination of the spinal cord. Meningeal and plexal infiltrations were not mentioned, nor were lesions of other organs described.

In the case of Viets and Warren (14) in which death occurred on the fourteenth day, the diagnosis also lacked confirmation by virus isolation or development of protective antibodies. Like some of the foregoing cases, it presented more encephalitic lesions than have been usual in inoculated monkeys. There was infiltration by small and fewer large lymphocytes and few endothelial cells in the congested, edematous meninges and in sheaths of perforating vessels and of larger vessels in the cortical white substance. Paravascular gliosis occurred there, and more extensively in the midbrain. Some perivascular hemorrhage was noted, as well as some leucocyte infiltration of vessel walls and some macrophages in glia foci. Warren's oxyphil inclusion bodies occurred apparently in the pigmented neurons of the substantia nigra. I have seen similar oxyphil granules in pigmented neurons of the locus coeruleus in young monkeys.

Aside from the note of pulmonary congestion and edema and of slight cystitis in the gross protocol, the organs were not described.

In the case reported by Machella, Weinberger and Lippincott (15), the diagnosis also rested on clinical findings alone, since virus was not recovered from the inoculated guinea pigs. This case, in which death occurred thirty days after onset, presented meningeal lymphocyte infiltration and fibroblast proliferation, with focal hemorrhage and hemosiderotic macrophage infiltration and patches of organizing fibrin on the base. Other conditions noted were ependymal desquamation and pronounced subependymal gliosis and perivascular lymphocyte infiltration; intraventricular exudate of fibrin, red cells, chorioidal epithelium, macrophages, and various leucocytes; and dense inflammatory cell infiltration of chorioidal villi with hemorrhage and distal epithelial necrosis. Otherwise no important parenchymal changes were noted and lesions of other viscera were not mentioned.

The cerebral lesions in this case appear to mimic those of the inoculated monkeys rather closely.

Three further autopsies were reported as acute lymphocytic choriomeningitis by Silcott and Neubuerger (16), again without etiologic confirmation by virus isoation or serum protection tests.

The first, quite acute, case presented a chiefly lymphocytic meningeal infiltration, more pronounced about vessels and on the brain stem, with very moderate subcortical cerebral perivascular lymphocyte infiltration, and some "glia stars" in cerebellum, olives, substantia nigra, and (fewer) cerebral cortex. The chorioid plexus was normal. Otherwise there were confluent bilateral bronchopneumonia of the lower lobes, arteriosclerosis, cardiac hypertrophy, moderate nephrosclerosis, and prostatic hypertrophy.

The second case, fatal in twenty-two days after a febrile illness with meningeal signs and symptoms, coma, and pleocytosis, presented some cerebral atrophy (1140 gm.), multiple areas of cystic softening in pons, thalamus, and internal capsule, focal hemorrhage, and pronounced atherosclerosis of basal arteries. Histologically there was a meningo-encephalitis: nodular glioses, petechiae, and much perivascular lymphocyte infiltration, especially in pons, locus coeruleus, and substantia nigra, and slight neuronal swelling and partial tigrolysis. Fibrous thickening of chorioidal villi and leptomeningeal lymphocyte infiltration completed the picture. Lesions of other organs were not mentioned.

Case 3 was clinically diagnosed as lymphocytic choriomeningitis but without further details. The autopsy revealed arteriosclerosis and gross cerebral atrophy, with moderate fibrosis and patchy lymphocyte infiltration of meninges, some perivascular lymphocyte infiltration, focal gliosis, and slight cell loss in the substantia nigra and the locus coeruleus, elsewhere essentially no lesions. The other viscera presented bronchiectasis, arteriosclerosis, and nephrosclerosis as the important anatomic findings.

The validity of these three cases as lymphocytic choriomeningitis is at least questionable.

There remain the apparently valid cases of Barker and Ford (17) and of Baker (18). In the former a fairly typical clinical attack was confirmed by isolation of the virus from spinal fluid, and on convalescence a motor and sensory paralysis of the lower extremities developed. Surgical exploration revealed a chronic fibrous spinal arachnoiditis, which was temporarily relieved by the decompression.

In Baker's case (18) death occurred after an illness of nine years duration. High titers of protective antibodies were found in the patient's blood serum at the first month and at the fifth year. There was gradual mental and neurological deterioration until death from aspiration pneumonia slightly over nine years from onset. At autopsy the brain presented general meningeal fibrosis and infiltration by lymphocytes, plasma cells, histiocytes, and perivascular phagocytes and lymphocytes. These changes were extensive over the brain stem, which showed relatively slight parenchymal alterations. The cerebral cortex presented marginal gliosis, vascular mural thickening and hyalinization, and cell pycnosis. Mononuclear cell infiltration of vessel sheaths was observed, and in the white substance there was extensive diffuse and focal demyelination, partly perivascular. About vessels there were also necrosis, cellular infiltration, and accumulation of phagocytic macrophages. In the cerebellum Purkinje cells were much reduced in numbers.

While the fact of infection with the virus is well established in this case, the process in the brain is rather that of a postinfection encephalomyelitis of the "isoallergic" type, such as one sees after antirabic vaccine, smallpox vaccination, measles, and the like. It seems probable that cases 7 and 8 of Howard's series (9) may be of this nature as well.

Inoculated monkeys (7, 11, 19, 20) have presented meningeal infiltration by lymphocytes and few other mononuclear cells. Plexal infiltration has been quite variable in extent and severity, from focal, purely lymphocytic, to diffuse, mixed lymphocytic, plasma-cell, and macrophage, with ventricular exudates of serum, fibrin, red corpuscles, a few neutrophils, many lymphocytes, macrophages, and chorioidal epithelial cells. Though inoculations were usually intracerebral, parenchymal vessel sheath infiltration was infrequent and focal gliosis rare.

Guinea pigs (11, 20, 21, 22, 24, 25) have presented similar but generally less pronounced meningoplexal reactions. In rats (19, 20, 24), similar reactions have been observed. Findlay and Stern (19) noted a higher proportion of polymorphonuclears in the exudate in rats than in other species. Kasahara, Hamano, and Yamada (20, 24) thought the reaction less severe in rats than in mice.

Most of the observations published have been on intracerebrally inoculated mice (4, 11, 19, 20, 22, 23, 26, 27, 28, 29). In these, meningeal exudates have been chiefly lymphocytic, with fewer macrophages and leucocytes, more pronounced on the base, in major fissures, and around the brain stem. Plexal infiltration was frequent, though inconstant, usually purely lymphocytic, and more pronounced in the third and fourth than in lateral ventricles. Both meningeal and plexal reactions were spare on the third to the fifth day after inoculation, and reached a maximum on the sixth to the ninth day (29). Intraventricular exudates were present in an increasing proportion (1/5, rising to 1/2) of the mice from the sixth to the ninth day, receding thereafter like the rest of the process. During the sixth to the ninth day period of maximal meningoplexal involvement there was a slight, less often moderate, lymphocyte infiltration of perforating and subependymal vessel sheaths, and, rarely, foci of cellular gliosis were found.

After noncerebral inoculation of mice (29), meningeal and plexal infiltration was often distinctly focal, absent in some animals, even maximal in intensity in some others, particularly with one certain virus strain (1650). Intraventricular exudation was strikingly infrequent.

Summing up, it appears that the meningoplexal infiltration by lymphoid and smaller numbers of other cells, with invasion of some cerebral vessel sheaths and occasional focal glioses, may be considered a direct virus effect, and most of the human autopsy cases have presented lesions of this general nature. Others have presented definitely intercurrent processes, or, as in Riggs's, Howard's, and Baker's cases, manifestations of the necrosing demyelinative type.

Except that one notes in the gross descriptions of several of the published human cases the presence of bronchopneumonia, noncerebral lesions in man have been conspicuous by their absence from the publications.

Fairly early in the studies of the virus of lymphocytic choriomeningitis, it became apparent that many healthy persons, without record of any past disease suggesting aseptic meningitis, possess protective antibodies against this virus in their blood serum (Armstrong [30]). Wooley, Armstrong, and Onstott (31) recorded such antibodies in 10 percent of a series of 1195 sera, contrasting with 17 (32 percent) of 53 sera from aseptic meningitis cases. Wooley, Stimpert, Kessel, and Armstrong (32) found protective antibodies in sera of healthy laboratory attendants. They recorded isolation of the virus from the blood of a laboratory attendant who was suffering from an influenza-like syndrome, without meningeal signs.

One of Howard's cases (9) from which virus was isolated presented no clinical signs of meningitis, though the spinal-fluid cell count reached 15 per cu. mm. Lépine, Mollaret, and Kreis (33) produced febrile illnesses of influenza-like nature by therapeutic inoculation of neurologic cases with mouse virus. These illnesses lasted from a few days up to three weeks, and in about half, meningeal signs were absent.

In Sautter's illness following laboratory infection (34), there was first a grippe-like syndrome which subsided in nine or ten days, followed by a second febrile attack from the thirteenth to the seventeenth day, during which she had meningeal symptoms. Virus was recovered.

Two members of the staff of this Institute have suffered from influenza-like illnesses. Their sera taken before the illnesses in question did not contain protective antibodies; after the illness these were present. In the first of these cases (35), virus was recovered from blood taken on the fifth day of illness. In the other (*KME*), the nature of the illness was not suspected until after recovery, and stored samples of the patient's serum revealed the story.

Aside from the pneumonias present in most of the fatal human cases, the presence or absence of visceral lesions has been ignored by most of the reports, and only the cases of Smadel *et al.* were fatal before the appearance of meningitic clinical signs and symptoms.

Studies of inoculated experimental animals have been made by Rivers and Scott (22), Traub (23, 26), Findlay, Alcock, and Stern (11), Findlay and Stern (19), Lépine and Sautter (27), Lépine, Kreis, and Sautter (28), Kasahara, Yamada, and Hamano (24), Kasahara, Hamano, and Yamada (20), Perrin and Steinhaus (25), and Shwartzman (36), as well as by myself and Armstrong (4, 7, 21, 29). These lesions I have considered in detail in the last cited paper, and will only attempt to summarize here.

Infiltrations which are best characterized as interstitial in the more highly vascular organs, and perivascular in the less vascular tissues, composed largely of lymphocytes, but including also, on occasion, plasma cells, monocytes or macrophages, and even a few polymorphonuclear leucocytes, have been described with variable frequency in almost every organ which has been studied histologically. It should be noted that the principal exceptions to this series are the lymphoid organs—the thymus, spleen, lymph nodes, and bone marrow—where lymphocytes or morphologically similar cells constitute an important part of the normal tissue structure. Such infiltrations have been found in all of the species studied—mice, rats, guinea pigs, and monkeys—with roughly comparable frequencies and intensities for the several organs, and with no great discrepancies among the various authors. Intensities of these reactions, where studied by the same author, have been found to vary according to the infecting virus strain, and have shown lesser frequencies and intensities in some organs after intracerebral than after other routes of infection or inoculation. When studied in relation to time from inoculation, these infiltrations appear later in the viscera after intracerebral inoculation, and later in the brain and meninges after noncerebral injection than conversely. These infiltrations seem to appear about 4 to 6 days after inoculation and increase in frequency and density well into the convalescence period. In fact, quite severe renal infiltrations was noted in mice 90 to 225 days after infection by Traub (26), and I (7) have noted meningeal lymphocyte infiltration in monkeys as late as 81 days, epididymal at 55 days, renal at 7 months, after inoculation.

In solid viscera the more striking lymphoid cell infiltrations have occurred in the renal pelvis and cortex in mice (19, 23, 26, 29, 36), rats (19), guinea pigs (21, 25), and monkeys (7, 11, 19); in the epididymis of monkeys (7) and less often mice (29), rarely guinea pigs (21); in the liver in mice (11, 19, 23, 27, 29, 36), guinea pigs (11, 19, 21, 23, 25), and monkeys (7, 11); and in the salivary gland and the pancreas in mice (19, 29), but infrequently in monkeys (7) or guinea pigs (25).

In addition to these infiltrations, there is often in mice an exudative serous pleurisy and peritonitis, with more or less profuse infiltrations of mediastinal and omental or mesenteric fatty tissues, proliferation and exfoliation of mesothelium, and serosanguinofibrinous exudates containing lymphoid cells, monocytes, and fewer leucocytes. Similar, though less striking, reactions were observed in monkeys (7) and guinea pigs (21, 25).

Fatty degeneration of liver and kidneys appears in mice at the third or fourth day and persists into the third week (11, 29). It has been observed also in the liver of guinea pigs (11, 19, 21, 23, 25) and monkeys (7, 11).

Focal coagulation necrosis, hyaline and necrotic cellular thrombi, and granulomatous replacement of these foci, we described in the mouse liver (29) between the fifth and ninth days, most often on the sixth and seventh. Similar lesions were seen also in guinea pigs. Necroses were described also by Findlay and Stern, by Traub, by Rivers and Scott, and by Shwartzman, in mice; by Findlay and coworkers, by Traub, and by Perrin and Steinhaus, in guinea pigs; by us and by Findlay, Alcock, and Stern, in monkeys. Focal necrosis of similar type is also noted less often in the adrenal cortex in mice (29) and (rarely) monkeys (7), and in the corpora lutea of mice (29). Areas of necrosis, hemorrhage, and serofibrinous exudate have been noted in lymph nodes, spleen, and, less often, bone marrow of mice, but not of guinea pigs or monkeys. Diffuse thymic lymphocyte depletion with karyorrhexis and phagocytosis were seen in mice (29) and guinea pigs (25).

CONCLUSIONS

Altogether the experimental pathology points to widespread generalization of the virus throughout the viscera as well as the central nervous system, with injuries of greater or less extent to these viscera occurring maximally about six or seven days after infection, and inflammatory reactions which apparently persist well into the convalescence and recovery periods.

Virus studies by Armstrong, Traub, Findlay and co-workers, and others have demonstrated this postulated wide distribution of the virus, and Armstrong and Traub have shown its long persistence after apparent convalescence. This last would appear to match with the long persistence of inflammatory lesions noted by us and by Traub.

REFERENCES

1. Blau, A., A case of serous meningoencephalitis, with autopsy report, *Arch. Otol.*, 1907, 36:432.
2. Beneke, R., Zur Ätiologie und Histogenese der Meningitis serosa cerebralis, *Arch. f. klin. Chir.*, 1934, 179:327.
3. Rizzo, C., Considerazzioni sulle meningiti asettiche sperimentali, *Riv. di Patol. nerv. e. ment.*, 1935, 46:373.
4. Armstrong, C., and R. D. Lillie, Experimental lymphocytic choriomeningitis of monkeys and mice produced by a virus encountered in studies of the 1933 St. Louis encephalitis epidemic, *Pub. Health Rep.*, 1934, 49:1019.
5. Margulis, M. S., Zur Nosographie und Pathogenese der akuten serösen Meningitiden, *Deut. Ztschr. Nervenheilk.*, 1927, 97:179.
6. McCordock, H. A., W. Collier, and S. H. Gray, The pathologic changes of the St. Louis type of acute encephalitis, *J.A.M.A.*, 1934, 103:822.
7. Lillie, R. D., Pathologic histology of lymphocytic choriomeningitis in monkeys, *Pub. Health Rep.*, 1936, 51:303.
8. Smadel, J. E., R. H. Green, R. M. Paltauf, and T. A. Gonzales, Lymphocytic choriomeningitis: Two human fatalities following an unusual febrile illness, *Proc. Soc. Exp. Biol. & Med.*, 1942, 49:683.
9. Howard, M. E., Infection with the virus of lymphocytic choriomeningitis in man, *Yale J. Biol. & Med.*, 1940, 13:161.
10. MacCallum, F. O., and G. M. Findlay, Lymphocytic choriomeningitis, *Lancet*, 1939, 1:1370.
11. Findlay, G. M., N. S. Alcock, and R. O. Stern, The virus aetiology of one form of lymphocytic meningitis, *Lancet*, 1936, 1:650.
12. Riggs, Helen E., Pathologic changes in a case of fatal lymphocytic meningo-encephalitis, *Arch. Neur. Psych.*, 1936, 36:1394.
13. Noone, E. L., Epidemic lymphocytic meningo-encephalitis, *Arch. Neur. Psych.*, 1936, 36:1393.
14. Viets, H. R., and S. Warren, Acute lymphocytic meningitis, *J.A.M.A.*, 1937, 108:357.

15. Machella, T. E., L. M. Weinberger, and S. W. Lippincott, Lymphocytic choriomeningitis. Report of a fatal case with autopsy findings. *Am. J. Med. Sci.*, 1939, 197:617.
16. Silcott, W. L., and K. Neubuerger, Acute lymphocytic choriomeningitis. Report of three cases with histopathologic findings, *Am. J. Med. Sci.*, 1940, 200:253.
17. Barker, L. F., and F. R. Ford, Chronic arachnoiditis obliterating the spinal subarachnoid space, *J.A.M.A.* 1937, 109:785.
18. Baker, A. B., Chronic lymphocytic choriomeningitis, *J. Neuropath. & Exp. Neurol.*, 1947, 6:253.
19. Findlay, G. M., and R. O. Stern, Pathological changes due to infection with the virus of lymphocytic choriomeningitis, *J. Path. & Bact.*, 1936, 43:327.
20. Kasahara, S., R. Hamano, and R. Yamada, Choriomeningitis virus isolated in the course of experimental studies on epidemic encephalitis, *Kitasato Arch. Exp. Med.*, 1939, 16:24.
21. Lillie, R. D., and C. Armstrong, Pathologic reaction to the virus of lymphocytic choriomeningitis in guinea pigs, *Pub. Health Rep.* 1944, 59:1391.
22. Rivers, T. M., and T. F. McN. Scott, Meningitis in man caused by a filterable vivrus. II: Identification of the etiological agent, *J. Exp. Med.*, 1936, 63:415.
23. Traub, E., An epidemic in a mouse colony due to the virus of acute lymphocytic choriomeningitis, *J. Exp. Med.*, 1936, 63:533.
24. Kasahara, S., R. Yamada, and R. Hamano, Chorioidal meningitis virus isolated during the study of experimental encephalitis (abstract), *Kitasato Arch. Exp. Med.*, 1937, 14:7.
25. Perrin, T. L., and E. A. Steinhaus, Pathologic reaction in guinea pigs to the Humphrey's virus strain, *Pub. Health Rep.*, 1944, 59:1603.
26. Traub, E., Persistence of lymphocytic choriomeningitis virus in immune animals and its relation to immunity, *J. Exp. Med.*, 1936, 63:847.
27. Lépine, P., and V. Sautter, Existence en France du virus murin de la chorio-méningite lymphocytaire, *Compt. rend. Acad. Sci.*, 1936, 202: 1624.
28. Lépine, P., B. Kreis, and V. Sautter, Sensibilité de la souris, du cobaye et du rat au virus parisien de la chorio-méningite lymphocytaire, *Compt. rend. Soc. Biol.*, 1937, 124:420.
29. Lillie, R. D., and Charles Armstrong, Pathology of lymphocytic choriomeningitis in mice, *Arch. Path.*, 1945, 40:141.
30. Armstrong, Charles, Acute lymphocytic choriomeningitis, experimental considerations, *Arch. Neurol. & Psychiat.*, 1936, 36:1395.
31. Wooley, J. G., C. Armstrong, and R. Onstott, The occurrence in the sera of man and monkeys of protective antibodies against the virus of lymphocytic meningitis as determined by the serum-virus protection tests in mice, *Pub. Health Rep.* 1937, 52:1105.

32. Wooley, J. G., F. D. Stimpert, J. F. Kessel, and C. Armstrong, A study of human sera antibodies capable of neutralizing the virus of lymphocytic choriomeningitis, *Pub. Health Rep.*, 1939, 54:938.
33. Lépine, P., P. Mollaret, and B. Kreis, Réceptivité de l'homme au virus murin de la chorioméningite lymphocytaire. Reproduction expérimentale de la méningite lymphocytaire bénigne, *Comptes rend. Acad. Sci.*, 1937, 204:1846.
34. Lépine, P., and V. Sautter, Contamination de laboratoire avec le virus de la chorioméningite lymphocytaire, *Ann. Inst. Pasteur*, 1938, 61:519.
35. Armstrong, C., and J. W. Hornibrook, Choriomeningitis virus infection without central nervous system manifestations. Report of a case, *Pub. Health Rep.*, 1941, 56:907.
36. Shwartzman, G., Alterations in pathogenesis of experimental lymphocytic choriomeningitis caused by prepassage of the virus through heterologous host. *J. Immunol.* 1946, 54:293.

Chapter 14

THE PATHOLOGY OF SOME VIRAL ENCEPHALITIDES[1]

By ABNER WOLF, *Departments of Pathology and Neurology, Columbia University College of Physicians and Surgeons and the Neurological Institute of New York*

THE VIRAL ENCEPHALITIDES to be discussed may be subdivided for ease of presentation into three main groups. The first is represented by von Economo's, or lethargic encephalitis and rabies. Lethargic encephalitis involves the brain stem most severely and is a subacute or chronic process. Its lesions are most often concentrated at the rostral extremity of the brain stem in contrast to rabies, an acute encephalomyelitis, in which they are more intense at its caudal end. The second group is composed essentially of the arthropod-borne encephalitides, a series of acute infections transmitted to man chiefly by the bite of insects. In these, the lesions are found in all parts of the central nervous system, with the brunt of the attack being borne by the basal structures of the brain and by the cerebral cortex. This group is represented here by St. Louis, Eastern and Western equine encephalomyelitis and Japanese B encephalitis, and includes among others the presently extinct Australian X disease, South American, or Venezuelan encephalomyelitis, and Russian spring-forest encephalitis. The third group is composed of herpes simplex and inclusion encephalitis, in which the cerebral cortex suffers most, so that mental symptoms may be prominent, with the cerebral white matter and basal ganglia being serious sufferers, as well. The first is an acute and the second an acute, subacute or a chronic relapsing condition

[1] This description of the comparative pathology of a series of representative viral encephalitides has been made possible by the generous contribution of material by many of my colleagues in Boston, Washington, D. C., Chicago, Cincinnati, St. Louis, New Orleans, and Vienna. To name only a few, Drs. Haymaker, Dunlap, Gray, Russel, Farber, Weil, Baker and Cauders contributed much valuable material, some still in the process of publication, and Dr. Haymaker very kindly permitted me to read two manuscripts in press. I am deeply grateful for the opportunity to study and compare this material, to draw my own conclusions, and report upon them. No diseases are described which I did not have the opportunity to see and study for myself.

of great interest. In the first two groups the spinal cord is involved to a variable degree, and in the third group, little, if at all.

When the encephalitides are viewed in this fashion, we find that one end of the brain, its caudal extremity, the brain stem, suffers most in conditions in group one, which includes lethargic encephalitis, and that the rostral extremity of the brain, represented by the cerebral cortex, suffers most in group three, herpes simplex and inclusion encephalitis. This is a conscious oversimplification, with full knowledge of the wide overlapping of the appearance and distribution of the lesions in the various encephalitides.

In two of the diseases under consideration here, von Economo's and inclusion encephalitis, the virus etiology of the condition has not been established. The suspicion is very strong in each, however, that a virus is the causative agent.

GROUP ONE

Rabies. Although rabies may have a long incubation period, during which the virus travels from the site of the bite of the rabid animal along a peripheral nerve to the central nervous system, there is an acute and highly fatal encephalomyelitis when it reaches and is able to infect the brain and spinal cord. There are usually edema and hyperemia of these structures, which are most marked in the medulla and the cervical spinal cord. Histologically, the leptomeninges are congested and show a mild infiltration by lymphocytes near the focal parenchymal lesions. The medulla exhibits the most intense lesions. Here there are hyperemia, occasional perivascular hemorrhages, degeneration of nerve cells in the cranial nerve nuclei associated with focal inflammatory changes, and a localized extension of the process into near-by white matter, where axons and myelin sheaths may occasionally break down. On the whole, the emphasis of the abnormal changes is on foci in the gray matter. The process is also severe in the pons and the midbrain and frequently in the thalamus. The hippocampal cortex suffers more than other portions of the cerebral cortex, which on the whole tend to be spared. The gray horns and adjacent portions of the white columns of the spinal cord may be the site of advanced degenerative changes in some instances, with associated lesions in the dorsal ganglia, and there may be greater involvement on the side of, and in the cord segment corresponding to, the site of the bite.

The nerve cell changes lack any specificity and are variable in their character, except for the occurrence of specific cytoplasmic inclusions known as Negri bodies. These are rounded or oval, eosinophilic bodies lying within spaces in the protoplasm of a nerve cell and containing basophilic granules. They vary considerably in size, may be single or multiple, and occur not only in the body of the cell, but occasionally in its dendrites as well. Upon dissolution of the nerve cell, Negri bodies may be found free in the tissue. Negri bodies are encountered in the hippocampus, in the pyramidal layer of other portions of the cerebral cortex, in Purkinje cells, in the large nerve cells of the basal ganglia and cranial nerve nuclei, the dorsal root ganglia, the ganglionic layer of the retina, and the ganglia of the sympathetic nervous system. There are moderate inflammatory phenomena, evidenced as perivascular and milder focal parenchymal infiltration by lymphocytes and fewer polymorphonuclear leucocytes. The latter may occasionally predominate. These accompany the degenerative changes in the nerve cells but may be present in some foci where no obvious changes in the nerve cells are observable. Conversely, Negri bodies may be encountered in groups of nerve cells which appear relatively well preserved, in the absence of local inflammatory changes. As nerve cells break down, there may be an initial phagocytosis by polymorphonuclear leucocytes. This neuronophagia by hematogenous elements is rapidly followed by microglial activation and phagocyte formation. Clusters of such hematogenous and microglial phagocytes are the Babès nodules, once mistakenly thought to be specific. Equivalent neuronophagia may occur in the dorsal ganglia, with the capsular cells proliferating in place of the microglia. In the focal lesions in the central nervous system, proliferating microglia are present in moderate numbers among the affected nerve cells and about the blood vessels showing inflammatory changes. These cells are usually in an intermediate stage of hypertrophy.

Lethargic encephalitis. In von Economo's, or lethargic, encephalitis, the second example of group one, the upper, or cephalic, end of the brain stem is the chief site of the disease process. Grossly the brain frequently appears normal, although it may be somewhat congested. The disease affects primarily the midbrain, the walls of the third ventricle, and the basal ganglia, its impact being almost wholly upon the gray matter. From this center of involvement, which explains its cardinal symptoms, such as sleep disturbances, abnormalities of the eye movements, extrapyramidal motor disabilities, and vegetative disturbances, one may follow the process in attenuated form into the cerebral cortex, where it is often meager, and into the pons, medulla, and roof nuclei of the cerebellum, where it is more striking. Far less often the gray matter of the spinal cord is irregularly involved. The lesions are focal and are marked by perivascular and some parenchymal lymphocytic infiltration (Plate I, Fig. 1), with occasional plasma cells in accord with their subacute or chronic nature. There is local destruction of nerve cells, accompanied by microgliosis and a gradually developing astrocytosis. Although satellitosis and neuronophagia occur, diffuse microglial hypertrophy is seen within each focus of involvement. In some of the severer lesions a necrosis associated with liquefaction of the tissue may occur and microglial phagocytes may become abundant, but it is never as marked as in some of the conditions to be discussed below. The astrocytosis matures and glial scarring later marks the area of nerve cell destruction. In one of the most characteristically affected structures, the substantia nigra, this disappearance of nerve cells results in a gross blanching of the normally dark-brown nuclear strip. Occasionally one encounters some persistence of perivascular lymphocytic infiltration long after the initial, active phase of the disease is past, when the patient has developed signs of a postencephalitic Parkinson's syndrome, but this is uncommon. In view of the progressive development of symptoms in Parkinson's syndrome, such continuing inflammation has been attributed by some to a persistent, intermittent activity of the etiologic agent in the central nervous system. In the absence of any direct knowledge of the causative factor this is purely speculative.

GROUP TWO

In group two are the arthropod-borne encephalitides, marked by acute inflammation, rapid course, and rostral emphasis in location of the disease process, as compared to group one, in that the thalamus, basal ganglia, cerebral cortex, and in many, the cerebral white matter, as well, are extensively involved. The basal structures of the cerebrum

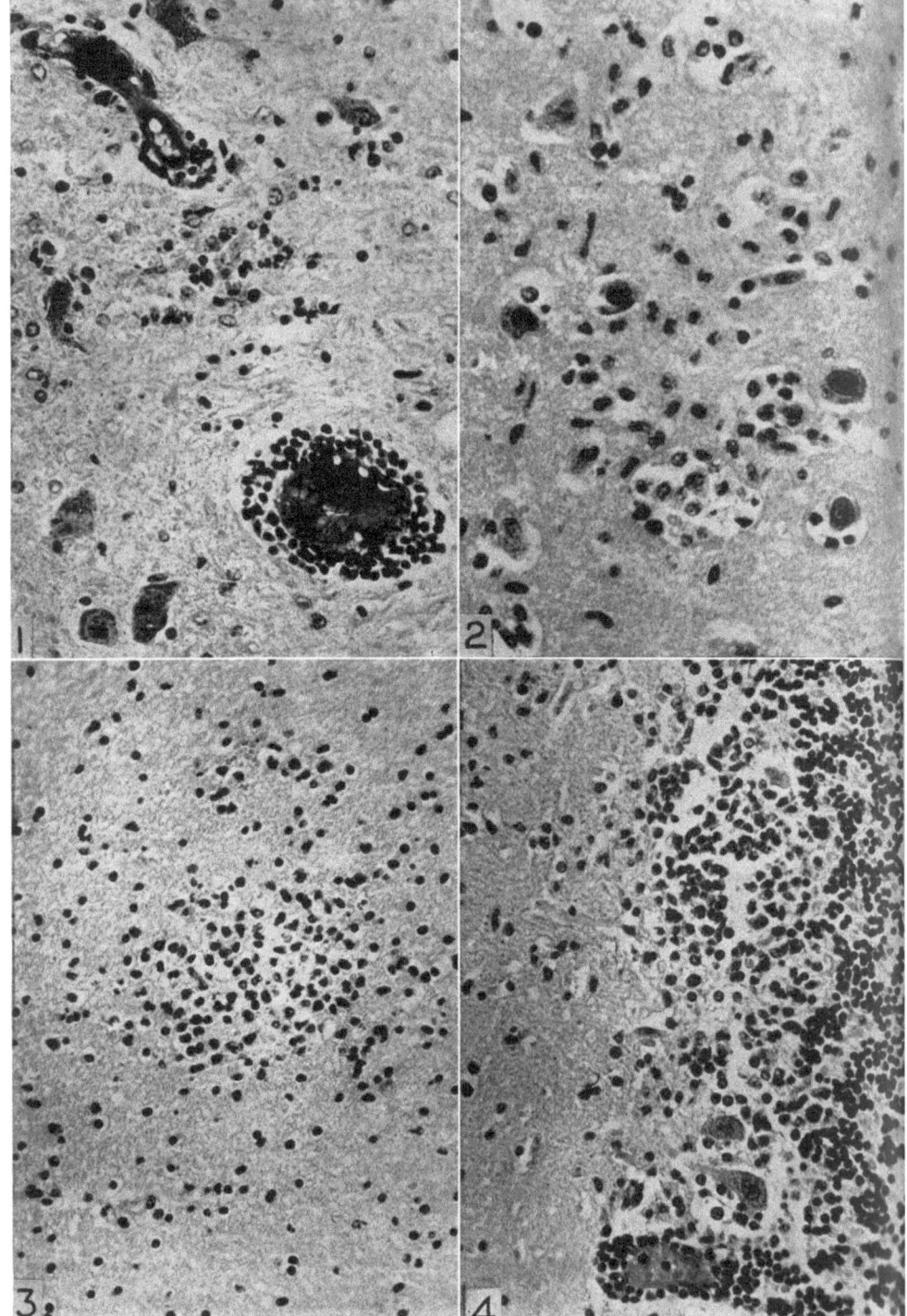

are the chief field of virus invasion, which is by way of the blood stream. The spinal cord is far more frequently and extensively affected than in group one, and the cerebellar cortex is involved, in some instances extensively so. Most often in children, but also in young adults and in the elderly, the lesions of the diseases in this group may result in widespread devastation of large areas of the cerebrum and lead to serious permanent neurological defects.

St. Louis encephalitis. This is one of the milder instances of this group of encephalomyelitides, in that focal necrosis of the tissue is far less commonly encountered and thus, if the patient recovers, permanent neurological sequelae are rare. Grossly, the brain may be normal in appearance, or somewhat congested with the hyperemia being patchy or diffuse. Histologically, lesions are found to be scattered from cerebral cortex to spinal cord, sparing neither the gray nor the white matter and predominating in the former. In general, the basal structures of the brain are the most intensely affected. Leptomeningeal infiltration is much more evident than in lethargic encephalitis, and is often marked by the presence of neutrophiles among the lymphocytes. Focal lesions in the gray matter (Plate I, Fig. 2) and white matter (Plate I, Fig. 3) consist of perivascular and parenchymal infiltration by neu-

---

PLATE I

FIGURE 1. EPIDEMIC ENCEPHALITIS. SUBSTANTIA NIGRA
Perivascular infiltration by lymphocytes. Disintegration and neuronophagia of nerve cell. Hematoxylin and eosin. Magnification = × 175.

FIGURE 2. ST. LOUIS ENCEPHALITIS. CEREBRAL CORTEX
Focal infiltration by polymorphonuclear neutrophiles with microglial activation. Hematoxylin and eosin. Magnification = × 175.

FIGURE 3. ST. LOUIS ENCEPHALITIS. CEREBRAL WHITE MATTER
Focal lesion showing microglial proliferation and infiltration by polymorphonuclear neutrophiles. Hematoxylin and eosin. Magnification = × 100.

FIGURE 4. ST. LOUIS ENCEPHALITIS. CEREBELLUM
Focal degeneration and neuronophagia of Purkinje cells. Diffuse and perivascular infiltration by lymphocytes and polymorphnuclear neutrophiles in Purkinje cell and molecular layers. Hematoxylin and eosin. Magnification = × 100.

trophiles and lymphocytes, with the former predominating at first (Plate I, Fig. 2) and the latter subsequently (Plate I, Fig. 4). This is associated with moderate focal microglial proliferation (Plate I, Fig. 3). Nerve cells may be anatomically intact in such areas or may show only mild signs of degeneration having no specific features. Occasionally there may be localized areas of necrosis of the tissue with more intense neutrophilic infiltration, and in such lesions all local nerve cells and their processes and sheaths and many neuroglial elements may succumb. Here microglial phagocytes gather. Such necrotizing lesions are relatively uncommon in this disease, as compared to their frequency in the conditions described below.

Eastern and Western equine encephalomyelitis. The second and third examples of group two are the American equinine encephalomyelitides. Here again, we are dealing with acute, rapidly progressive, blood-borne and arthropod-transmitted infections, widespread in the brain and spinal cord and affecting both gray and white matter, the former more severely. Once more, although the basal structures of the cerebrum are injured most by the respective viruses of these two diseases, the cerebral cortex and the white matter suffer regularly and extensively, as well. The brain stem and the spinal cord are commonly affected, and not infrequently the cerebellum is involved. Grossly, the brain may appear normal or be congested in the acute phase of the disease. Histologically, the leptomeninges are the site of an infiltration localized chiefly over underlying parenchymal inflammation and marked by neutrophiles early and lymphocytes later. Foci of perivascular and parenchymal inflammation of the same type are found widely disseminated throughout the associated gray and white matter with focal microglial proliferation (Plate II, Fig. 2), but here they are frequently the site of degeneration of nerve cells, myelin sheaths, axons, and glial cells. There may be total necrosis of all of the elements in such a focus with intense polymorphonuclear infiltration, so that the lesion may resemble a miliary abscess. In these there is usually a considerable admixture of newly formed microglial phagocytes (Plate II, Fig. 2). In the white matter, in myelin stains, such lesions have the appearance of sharply demarcated foci of demyelination (Plate II, Fig. 3), and in some that are less severe the axones may be partially preserved while the myelin sheaths have totally disappeared. Pale, sharply demarcated zones of acute degeneration, having a punched-out appearance (Plate II, Fig. 1), may be encountered chiefly in the gray matter of the cerebrum, and have been recently described from New Orleans. These are remarkable for their lack of inflammatory or glial response and are similar to lesions described recently by Zimmerman in Japanese B encephalitis. Some of the zones of degeneration in both the gray and the white matter may be more diffuse and frequently have a striking resemblance to lesions resulting from an interference with the local circulation, although no anatomical evidence of such circulatory disturbances can be detected. Such areas are edematous, and many fields of nerve cells in them are found to be undergoing ischemic necrosis with little or no regional inflammation. In such areas all structures eventually succumb, including the mesodermal elements. Phagecytosis, chiefly by activated microglial elements, occurs, and there is a marginal astrocytosis (Plate II, Fig. 4). Eventually cysts remain, lined by a modest wall of glial fibers, the whole process being accompanied by minimal inflammation. Both grossly and microscopically these lesions resemble progressively developing areas of encephalomalacia due to a circulatory abnormality; in the severer cases they result in irregularly atrophied brains showing considerable cavitation. In children calcification may occur in the malacic areas (Plate III, Fig. 1). Such intense degeneration is the cause of some of the profoundly incapacitating sequelae of these infections, more particularly in the young.

Japanese B encephalitis. The similarities between this disease and American equine encephalomyelitis are striking. The emphasis on destruction of cerebral cortex and basal ganglia is marked, and tissue liquefaction may be extreme. Zimmerman, in describing the gross appearance of the central nervous system in those dying within two weeks of the inception of symptoms, found few, if any, macroscopic changes in these acute cases. In some, focal congestion and clusters of petechial hemorrhages were seen in the cerebral cortex and in the basal ganglia, and these were few, inconstant, and variably distributed. Rarely there was focal blurring of the cerebellar cortical pattern, and congestion and discoloration of the gray matter of the spinal cord, as in poliomyelitis. In three patients who lived more than a month, there were widespread pale, sometimes finely granular and gritty, patches in the cerebral cortex and in the basilar nuclei of the cerebrum. They were larger in the latter, where they most often appeared in the globus

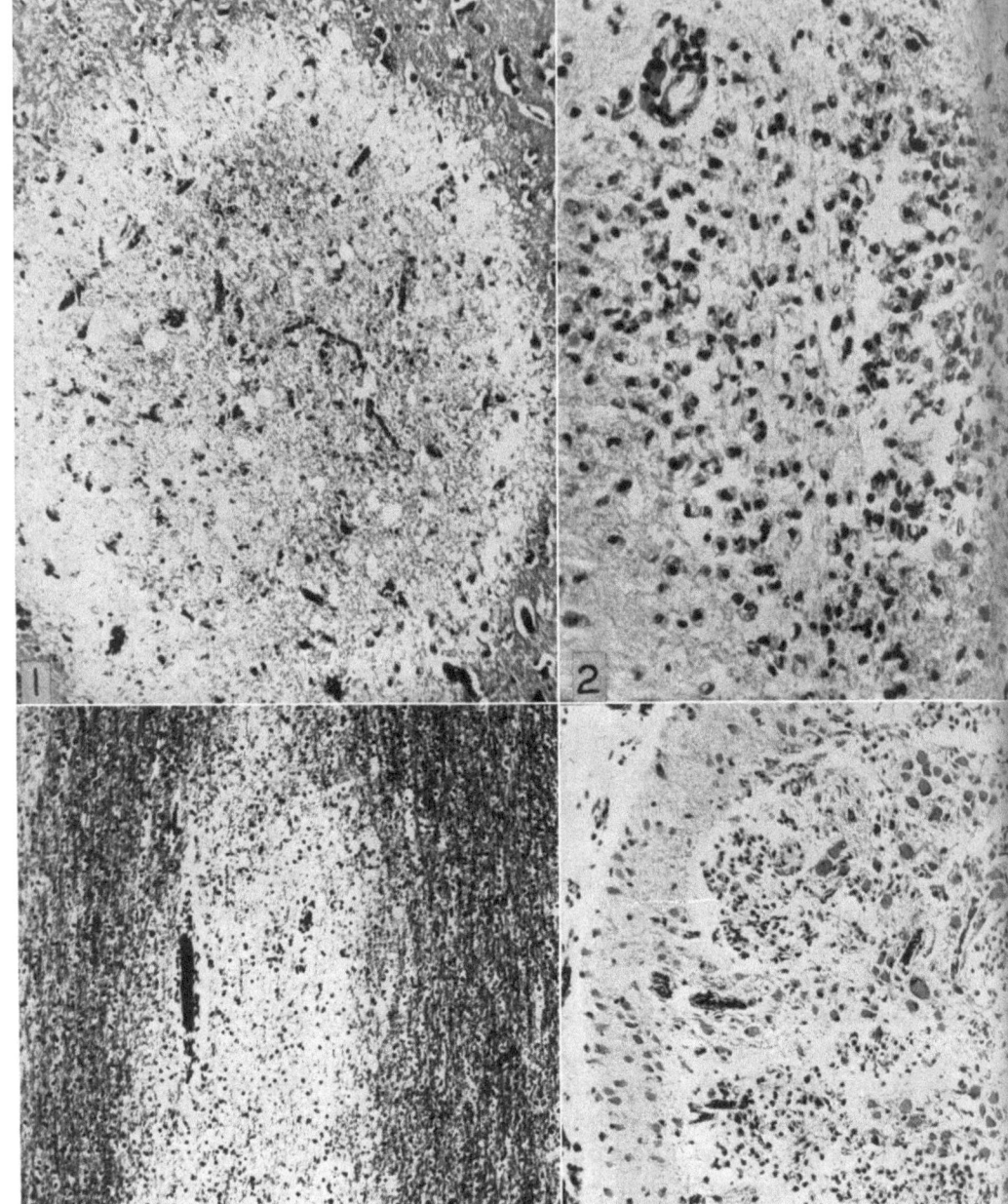

pallidus, thalamus, red nucleus, and substantia nigra. There were blurring of the cortical pattern of some cerebellar folia, tiny foci of brown discoloration of pontine and dentate nuclei, and, rarely, lack of clarity of the outlines of the gray matter in the spinal cord.

Histologically, there is mild lymphocytic infiltration of the leptomeninges. Small focal or larger diffuse areas of degeneration of nerve cells are encountered throughout the brain and spinal cord and are most conspicuous in the cerebral cortex and the basilar cerebral nuclei. These include a variety of cell changes, none of which are specific, and among which ischemic necrosis may be a striking feature, in some areas. Congestion, fresh perivascular hemorrhages, and mild or moderate perivascular infiltration by lymphocytes and occasional neutrophiles may accompany the neuronal changes or may be encountered independent of them. Neuronophagia by neutrophiles may be an early feature of the focal lesions. Here again, as in equine encephalomyelitis, neutrophiles are present early in these focal lesions and may be mixed with activated microglia to produce a highly cellular focus superficially resembling a miliary abscess (Plate III, Fig. 2). Punched-out areas of pallor in which nerve cells are markedly degenerated are described

---

PLATE II

FIGURE 1. EASTERN EQUINE ENCEPHALOMYELITIS. CEREBRAL CORTEX
Punched-out area of acute degeneration and pallor with little or no inflammation. Hematoxylin and eosin. Magnification = × 65.

FIGURE 2. WESTERN EQUINE ENCEPHALOMYELITIS. FOCAL NECROTIZING LESION IN CEREBRAL WHITE MATTER
Infiltration by polymorphonuclear neutrophiles and lymphocytes. Activation of microglia with the formation of large mononuclear phagocytes. Hematoxylin and eosin. Magnification = × 150.

FIGURE 3. EASTERN EQUINE ENCEPHALOMYELITIS. ACUTE, FOCAL, NECROTIZING LESION IN SUBCORTICAL WHITE MATTER SHOWING DEGENERATION OF MYELIN
Mahon. Magnification = × 55.

FIGURE 4. EASTERN EQUINE ENCEPHALOMYELITIS. CEREBRAL CORTEX
Infant dying two months after inception of illness. Inflammation has subsided. Obscuration of cortical architecture due to loss of nerve cells and many glial cells with cyst formation. Large mononuclear phagocytes in spaces with marginal astrocytosis. Hematoxylin and eosin. Magnification = × 65.

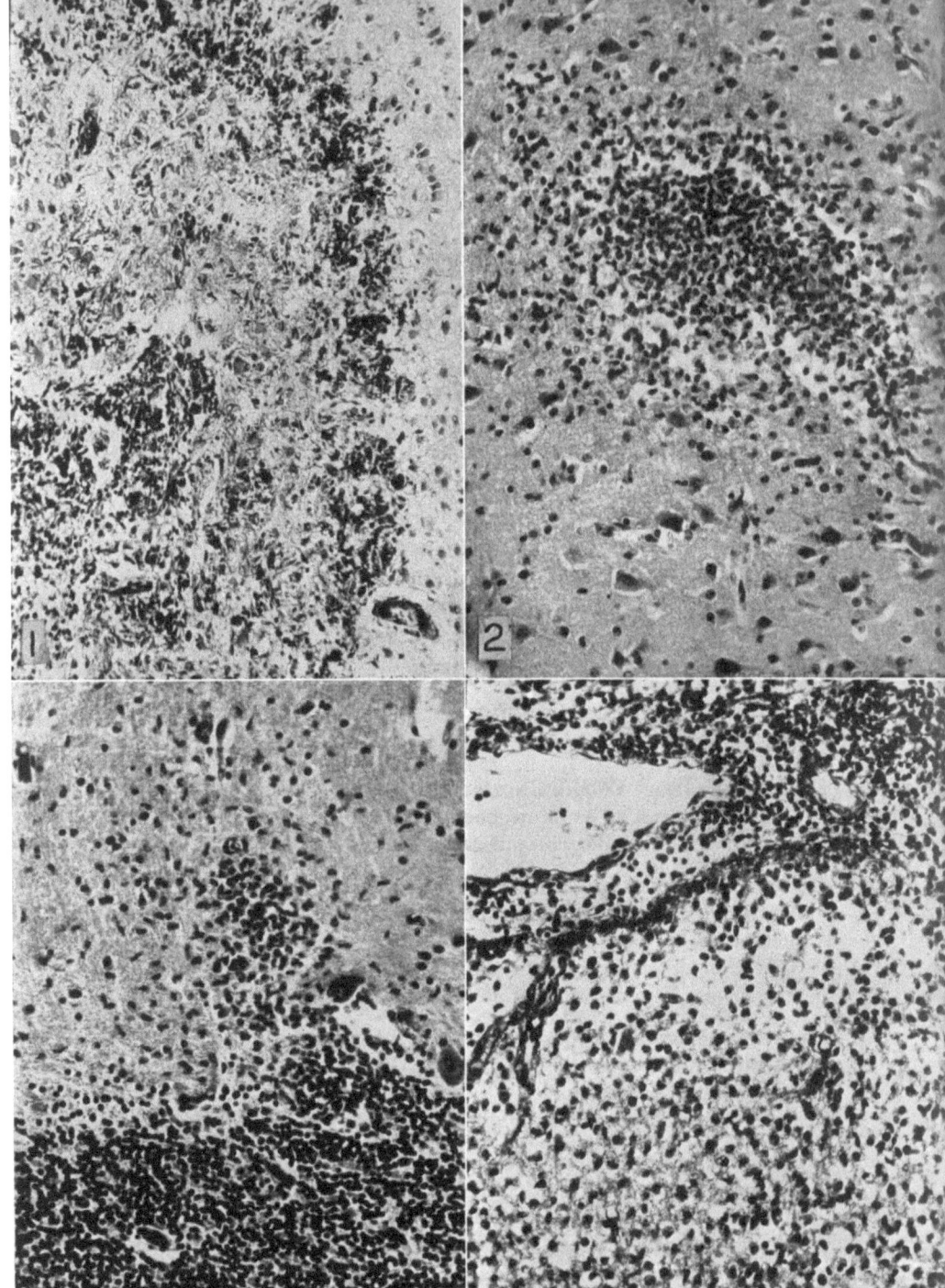

by Zimmerman as occurring primarily in the cerebral cortex. In these, as in the identical lesions described in equine encephalomyelitis, inflammation is absent or minimal and glial reaction lacking. As nerve cells disappear, the tissue becomes progressively more rarefied, loose-meshed, and lacy. Microglial proliferation and hypertrophy occur in nodular form as a satellitosis and a neuronophagia or are more diffuse in the individual focal lesions. As focal necrosis of the tissue occurs, large mononuclear phagocytes, chiefly of microglial origin, mingle with the neutrophiles and replace them. The frequent involvement of the cerebellar cortex, especially the destruction of Purkinje cells (Plate III, Fig. 3), combined with the often severe lesions in the gray matter of the spinal cord, have been compared to the findings in louping-ill in sheep. The major difference between Japanese B and the American equine encephalitides is the relatively slight involvement of white matter in the brain and spinal cord of the former, marked only by mild or moderate perivascular lymphocytic infiltration. In the surviving individual suffering from extensive necrotizing lesions, cystic areas of encephalomalacia like those described in equine encephalomyelitis are encountered. Zimmerman has demonstrated the occurrence of cal-

---

PLATE III

FIGURE 1. EASTERN EQUINE ENCEPHALOMYELITIS. CEREBRAL CORTEX
Infant dying two months after inception of illness. Extensive degeneration, gliosis, and calcification of cortex. Hematoxylin and eosin. Magnification = × 65.

FIGURE 2. JAPANESE B ENCEPHALITIS. CEREBRAL CORTEX
Focal, necrotizing, abscess-like lesion. Local destruction of neural and many glial elements with marked microglial proliferation and some polymorphonuclear infiltration. Hematoxylin and eosin. Magnification = × 75.

FIGURE 3. JAPANESE B ENCEPHALITIS. CEREBELLUM
Focal lesion in Purkinje cell and molecular layers marked by nerve cell degeneration, microglial proliferation and infiltration by lymphocytes. Hematoxylin and eosin. Magnification = × 65.

FIGURE 4. HERPES SIMPLEX ENCEPHALITIS. CEREBRAL CORTEX
Diffuse degeneration of upper layers of cerebral cortex with phagocyte formation and lymphocytic infiltration of leptomeninges and gray matter. Phloxin methylene blue. Magnification = × 75.

cification in such residual lesions in the young in Japanese B encephalitis.

GROUP THREE

The third group consists of herpes simplex and inclusion encephalitis. The virus etiology of the latter is not yet established, and some have suggested that inclusion encephalitis is one form of herpes simplex infection, but this is not proven. The two diseases—if they be two—are characterized by severe, diffuse, degenerative changes in the cerebral cortex and white matter and almost equally intense lesions in the basal structures of the cerebrum. The process becomes ever less marked as one examines the central nervous system in a caudad direction, and the cerebellum and spinal cord are little, if any, involved. Both diseases have affected children and young adults by preference in the small number of cases reported. Herpes simplex encephalitis is a fulminating, fatal infection by contrast with inclusion encephalitis, which is an acute, subacute, or chronic relapsing condition lasting from two months to seven years, the seven-year case being one of Haymaker's reported in a paper now in press. It is marked by repeated, severe exacerbations and by remissions, often of considerable duration. In both herpes simplex and inclusion encephalitis, there are cellular inclusions which are striking.

Herpes simplex encephalitis. The herpes simplex virus has many times been accused of being the causative agent of lethargic encephalitis. Such claims have been made on insufficient grounds and do not seem to be tenable. In the present decade Smith, Lennette, and Reames described the first authentic instances of herpes simplex infection of the central nervous system in man, and later Armstrong and thereafter Zarafonetis, Smadel, Adams, and Haymaker reported additional cases. Grossly, one may encounter focal areas of dusky discoloration, swollen, soft, and friable, which are studded with petechiae and are scattered through the brain but are seen most often in the cerebral cortex. When the brain is that of an infant, it may, as a whole, be soft and mushy far beyond what is usually encountered at this age. Histolgoically, the leptomeninges are found to be the site of a widespread leptomeningitis, most severe over cortical lesions. It is marked by lymphocytes, large mononuclear cells, plasma cells, and, less often, neutrophiles. Lesions in the neuraxis are severest at its rostral extremity and grow progressively less marked caudally. Thus the cerebral cortex is the site of the most numerous and most intense lesions, while the central white matter is less affected and most often in relation to the cortical changes. The basilar cerebral structures are less involved than either the cortex or the white matter. The rostral part of the brain stem is moderately affected, the caudal part and the cerebellum lightly, and the spinal cord not at all. The lesions in the cortex are varying-sized zones of intense degeneration and relatively mild inflammation (Plate III, Fig. 4). As a rule, it is more marked in the outer cortical layers, as if the process were sweeping in from the leptomeninges. The appearances are those of encephalomalacia due to a circulatory disturbance. Large numbers of nerve cells undergo ischemic necrosis, as well as other forms of acute degeneration. The tissue becomes rarefied, hosts of large mononuclear lipid-laden phagocytes flood the field, and capillaries show endothelial hyperplasia. The phagocytes appear to be microglial in origin and to originate from the blood vessel walls and leptomeninges as well. Satellitosis and neuronophagia are encountered. The blood vessel walls, perivascular spaces, and, to a lesser degree, the perivascular parenchyma are sparsely or moderately infiltrated with cells like those seen in the leptomeninges. Toward the margins of the cortical lesions fewer nerve cells are lost, and hypertrophied, elongated microglia cells in mid-activation are encountered. Here a mild astrocytosis is also seen. Sometimes segments of cortex may show widespread ischemic necrosis of their ganglion cells, with no local inflammation or almost none. Where the leptomeninges and superficial cerebral cortical layers are the site of masses of lipid-laden phagocytes, the line of demarcation between pia arachnoid and gray matter is often obscured. In descending order through the central white matter (Plate IV, Fig. 1) to the caudal portion of the brain stem, the lesions become more focal, less intense, and less necrotizing. Characteritic intranuclear inclusions are most common in the oligodendroglia (Plate IV, Fig. 3) and appear somewhat less frequently in nerve cells (Plate IV, Fig. 2). These are large, granular, sharply demarcated, and eosinophilic. They have a clear halo about them and are associated with margination of the basichromatin at the nuclear membrane. They are encountered most often in the cerebral cortex and white matter and are seen less often in the brain stem.

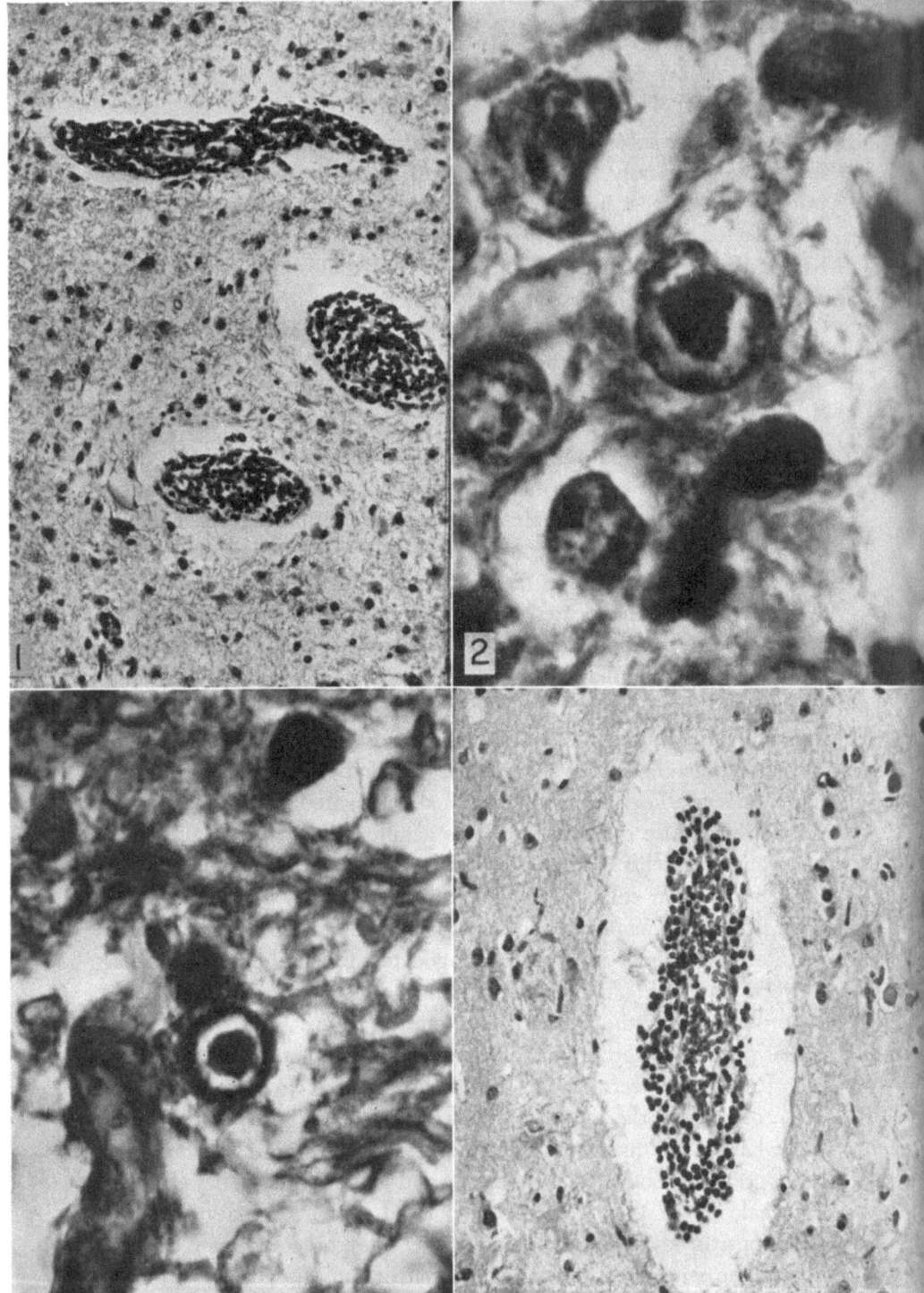

Inclusion encephalitis. Dawson described the first two instances of this disease in 1933 and 1934. This was followed by reports by Akelaitis and Zeldis (1942), Kinney (1942), Brain, Greenfield, and Russell (1943), and Swann (1943). A report by Malamud, Haymaker, and Pinkerton is now (1949) in press. This condition has not yet been proved to be due to a virus. In some instances, it is a remarkable relapsing disease in which symptoms may appear from time to time, with intervals during which the condition is stationary. Nearly all examples have occurred during the first two decades of life (in one case, at 21 years of age) and have been marked by striking mental symptoms and often by abnormal extrapyramidal motor phenomena. Again, as in the generally more acute herpes simplex encephalitis, the cerebral and subcortical white matter and, to a lesser degree, the basal cerebral structures are the sites of the most intense tissue destruction. The process extends throughout the neuraxis, involving the spinal cord. Inflammation is far less marked than in herpes simplex meningoencephalitis. There is a mild perivascular infiltration (Plate IV, Fig. 4) and some leptomeningeal infiltration by lymphocytes, but this is often absent. In the cerebral cortex, nerve cells are found in various stages

---

PLATE IV

FIGURE 1. HERPES SIMPLEX ENCEPHALITIS. CEREBRAL WHITE MATTER
Focal degeneration and astrocytosis with mural and perivascular infiltration by lymphocytes. Phloxin methylene blue. Magnification = × 50.

FIGURE 2. HERPES SIMPLEX ENCEPHALITIS. HIPPOCAMPAL CORTEX
Eosinophilic, granular, intranuclear inclusion in nerve cell with halo about inclusion and margination of basichromatin. Hematoxylin and eosin. Magnification = × 1100.

FIGURE 3. HERPES SIMPLEX ENCEPHALITIS. CENTRAL WHITE MATTER OF CEREBRUM
Eosinophilic intranuclear inclusion in oligodendrogial cell with halo about inclusion and margination of basochromatin. Hematoxylin and eosin. Magnification = × 1100.

FIGURE 4. INCLUSION ENCEPHALITIS. CEREBRAL CORTEX
Perivascular infiltration by lymphocytes. Diffuse degeneration of nerve cells; eosinophilic inclusions completely filling nuclei of some to right of blood vessel. Attendant astrocytosis. Hematoxylin and eosin. Magnification = × 75.

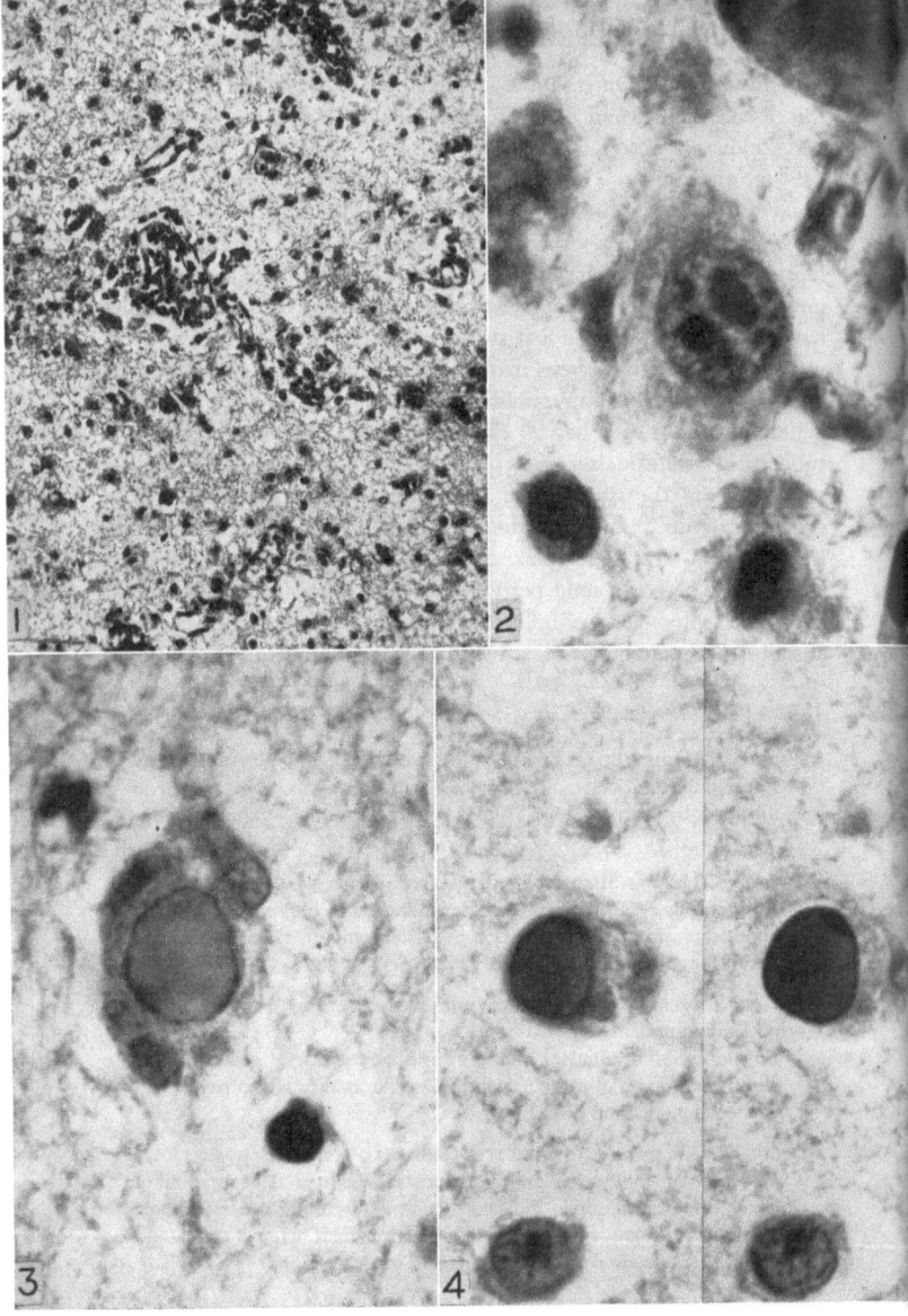

and forms of degeneration (Plate IV, Fig. 4). The microglia are activated and hypertrophy to form rod cells, and there is a diffuse, moderate astrocytosis (Plate IV, Fig. 4). There is a gradual loss of myelin sheaths in both the gray and the white matter and a lesser loss of axons with a similar glial reaction (Plate IV, Fig. 4). Zones of total necrosis occur but are far fewer than in herpes simplex encephalitis. Here all nerve and neuroglia cells and some of the mesodermal elements disappear, and there is a total demyelination, reproducing again the appearances of an encephalomalacia. All of these changes in the gray and white matter are quite diffuse. In addition, there are focal lesions, which are marked chiefly by clusters of proliferating microglia associated with relatively mild or no inflammation and relatively inconspicuous changes in the neural and neuroglial cells. In the older lesions, astrocytosis is prominent, and inflammation may in part persist and plasma cells be added to the lymphocytes. Many nerve cells have striking intranuclear, and some smaller and less clearly marked cytoplasmic, inclusions. The latter are usually seen in cells undergoing dissolution and always in the presence of intranuclear inclusions. Intranuclear inclusions are numerous but less frequent, in oligodendroglia. These intranuclear inclusions are usually single, and at first are granular and

---

PLATE V

FIGURE 1. INCLUSION ENCEPHALITIS. CEREBRAL WHITE MATTER
Diffuse degeneration and astrocytosis with slight perivascular infiltration by lymphocytes. Hematoxylin and eosin. Magnification = × 75.

FIGURE 2. INCLUSION ENCEPHALITIS. FOCAL LESION IN PONS
Eosinophilic intranuclear inclusion in nerve cell; nucleolus intact. Phloxin methylene blue. Magnification = × 1100.

FIGURE 3. INCLUSION ENCEPHALITIS. BASAL GANGLIA
Homogeneous inclusion completely filling nucleus of nerve cell. Note one large and two smaller cytoplasmic inclusion bodies. Phloxin methylene blue. Magnification = × 1100.

FIGURE 4. INCLUSION ENCEPHALITIS. CEREBRAL CORTEX
Two views of same nerve cell containing an intranuclear and a cytoplasmic inclusion body. Cytoplasmic inclusion sharply in focus on left and intranuclear inclusion clearly in focus on right. Phloxin methylene blue. Magnification = × 1100.

quite eosinophilic. In nerve cells the nucleoli are quite distinct and separate from them (Plate V, Fig. 2). Later, as they enlarge to fill the nucleus, they become homogeneous and turn a faint lavender (Plate V, Figs. 3, 4). There is margination of the basichromatin along the nuclear membrane, and at first, before they fill the nucleus, there is a clear halo about the inclusion. The cytoplasmic inclusions are less definite, are usually multiple, vary in size and shape, are hyaline and refractile, may be poorly defined, and have no clear space about them (Plate V, Figs. 3, 4). In one instance of long duration, Malamud, Haymaker, and Pinkerton have described widespread neurofibrillary degeneration in nerve cells resembling that recorded by Alzheimer in presenile dementia, but they encountered no pathological changes that were like senile plaques.

The increasing orientation of the more recently described virus infections of the central nervous system toward the cerebral cortex is but another indication of the special affinity of some viruses for certain cells, as exemplified by the tendency of the poliomyelitis virus to attack the motor cells, particularly those of the spinal cord. The fascinating problem of such specific localization can only be noted by the histopathologist. It may well be that some of the very valuable hints thrown out by my colleagues in this symposium may some day serve to explain part or all of this phenomenon.

REFERENCES

Rabies
Gamaleia, V., *Ann. Inst. Pasteur,* 1887, 1:63.
Babès, V., *Ann. Inst. Pasteur,* 1892, 2:374.
Van Gehuchten, A., and C. Nelis, *Le Nevraxe,* 1900, 1:79; *Presse med.,* 1900, 8:113.
Marinesco, G., *Soc. Biol. Paris,* 1909, 6:646; *C. R. Soc. Biol. Paris,* 1910, 68:898.
Marie, P., and C. Chatelin, *Bull. Acad. Med.,* 1919, 81:428.
Lowenburg, K., *Arch. Neurol. & Psychiat.,* 1928, 19:638.
Bassoe, P., and R. R. Grinker, *Arch. Neurol. & Psychiat.,* 1938, 23:1138.

Von Economo's, or Lethargic, Encephalitis
v. Economo, C., *Die Encephalitis lethargica* (Leipzig and Vienna, 1918; Vienna and Berlin, 1929).
Buzzard, E. F., and E. Farquhar, *Brain,* 1919, 42:305.
Creutzfeldt, H. G., *Ref. Z. Neur.,* 1920, 21:366.
Herzog, G., *Deut. Ztschr. Nervenheilk.,* 1921, 70:281.

Globus, J., and I. Strauss, *Arch. Neurol.*, 1922, 8:122.
Somogyi, J., *Z. Neur.*, 1924, 93:783.
Verga, P., and L. Uluhogian, *Rev. Pat. nerv.*, 1924, 29:370.
Spatz, H., *Zbl. Neur.*, 1925, 40:120.
Marinescu, D.-Baloi, *Arch. f. Psychiat.*, 1926, 76:704.
Cruchet, R. (Paris, 1928).

St. Louis Encephalitis
McCordock, H. A., W. Collier, S. H. Gray, *J. A. M. A.*, 1934, 103:822.
Weil, A., *Arch. Neurol. & Psychiat.*, 1934, 31:1139.

Eastern Equine Encephalomyelitis
Wesselhoeft, C., E. C. Smith, and C. F. Branch, *J.A.M.A.*, 1938, 111:1735.
Farber, S., A. Hill, M. L. Connerly, and J. H. Dingle, *J.A.M.A.*, 1940, 114:1725.

Western Equine Encephalomyelitis
Breslich, P. J., P. H. Rowe, and W. L. Lehman, *J.A.M.A.*, 1939, 113:1722.
Noran, H. H., and A. B. Baker, *Arch. Neurol. & Psychiat.*, 1942, 47:565; *J. Neuropath. & Exper. Neurol.*, 1945, 4:269.
Peers, J. H., *Arch. Path.*, 1942, 34:1050.

Japanese B Encephalitis
Taniguchi, T., M. Hosokawa, and S. Kuga, *Jap. J. Exp. Med.*, 1936, 14:185.
Hashimoto, H., M. Kudo, and K. Uraguchi, *J.A.M.A.*, 1936, 106:1266.
Zimmerman, H. M., *Am. J. Path.*, 1946, 22:965.
Haymaker, W., and A. B. Sabin, *Arch. Neurol. & Psychiat.*, 1947, 57:673.

Herpes Simplex Encephalitis
Smith, M. G., M. D. Lennette, and H. R. Reames, *Am. J. Path.*, 1941, 17:55.
Zarafonetis, C. J. D., J. E. Smadel, J. W. Adams, and W. Haymaker, *Am. J. Path.*, 1944, 20:429.
Whitman, L., and J. Warren, *J.A.M.A.*, 1946, 131:1408.
Haymaker, W., Presented at Annual Meeting of Amer. Assn. of Path. & Bact., March 13, 1948.

Inclusion Encephalitis
Dawson, J. R., *Am. J. Path.*, 1933, 9:7; *Arch. Neurol. & Psychiat.*, 1934, 31:685.
Akelaitis, A. J., and L. J. Zeldis, *Arch. Neurol. & Psychiat.*, 1942, 47:353.
Malamud, N., W. Haymaker, and H. Pinkerton, *Am. J. Path.*, 1949, in press.
Brain, W. R., J. G. Greenfield, and D. S. Russell, *Proc. Roy. Soc. Med.*, 1943, 36:319; *Brain*, 1948, 71:365.

Chapter 15

THE NATURE AND PATHOGENESIS OF NEURONAL CHANGES IN POLIOMYELITIS[1]

By Howard A. Howe, *Poliomyelitis Research Center, Department of Epidemiology, Johns Hopkins University*

It is the purpose of this review to demonstrate the neuronotropic character of poliomyelitis virus and to show how it conditions the fate of the central nervous system during active infection. In this respect, poliomyelitis appears to represent an extreme specialization which is matched only by that of rabies (1, 2). By comparison, the arthropod-borne encephalitic viruses are well toward the other end of the spectrum of the so-called neurotropes, since they circulate in the blood and appear to multiply in all the various elements of the central nervous system (3, 4, 5, 6). Most of the studies which I shall report on poliomyelitis have been carried out by Drs. Bodian, Mellors, Flexner, and myself in the laboratory at Johns Hopkins. Rhesus monkeys were used, but there is little reason to believe that the affinities of the virus for the central nervous system differ greatly in the chimpanzee or in man. True enough, these latter species are distinguished from the rhesus by the ability of the virus to multiply readily in the walls of the alimentary tract (7, 8). This fact is associated with alimentary susceptibility in the chimpanzee and possibly in man. These differences appear to reflect variations in resistance at the portal of entry, which could be hypothecated as due, either to differences in the rate at which virus is destroyed in the alimentary tract, and/or to a relative refractoriness of the epithelium and of other elements in the gut wall. Once the virus has entered the nervous system it appears to progress in identical fashion in all three hosts (8; 9, Chs. VI, VII; see also 10, 11).

Before coming to a consideration of the interaction between the virus and the individual neuron, I would like to mention some factors which limit the spread of the virus in the central nervous system. One of these is the differential susceptibility of different nerve centers, and

[1] The work reported in this article was supported in large part by the Commonwealth Fund and the National Foundation for Infantile Paralysis, Inc.

the other is the availability of nerve pathways along which the virus can travel. An example will suffice for each. There is a characteristic distribution of lesions which serves to distinguish poliomyelitis from other known neurotropic virus diseases in primates. One of its most notable features is the presence of lesions in the motor areas of the cortex, just anterior to the central sulcus (areas 4, 6, and 8), and their virtual absence from all other cerebral cortex. (Plate I, Fig. 1). That this represents more than the lack of suitable nerve connections, is shown by the fact that inoculations into the visual cortex of a rhesus monkey (area 17) produce no lesions here or elsewhere in the optic system, despite the fact that the animal contracts paralytic poliomyelitis and shows elsewhere many lesions of characteristic distribution. The difference in reaction between the motor and the visual cortex is clearly seen in the local response of these tissues to an inoculum placed in them. Whereas a radiating focus of lesions is seen in the motor area, the visual cortex shows only a foreign-body reaction (Plate 1, Figs. 2, 3). Although this pattern of refractoriness and susceptibility is doubtless due to chemical factors of which we have no present knowledge, it serves as a pathognomonic diagnostic feature which I should rate more characteristic of poliomyelitis than the lesions in the spinal cord (9, Chs. III, VI, VII; see also 12).

Accessibility also plays a role in determining the fate of certain centers in the central nervous system. For example, paralysis of the neck muscles is relatively uncommon in experimental animals inoculated by either intranasal or intracerebral routes, but it almost invariably occurs after inoculation into the vitreous of the eye. Here the route of invasion has been shown to be, not along the optic nerve but via the autonomic fibers of the oculomotor nerve to their cell bodies beneath the aqueduct of Sylvius (9, Ch. IV; 11). From here it is apparently a simple matter for the virus to reach the anterior horns of the upper cervical region, via the great coordinator of head and eye movements, the medial longitudinal fasciculus.

While the findings which I have just described can be explained only on the basis of neural transmission, we can narrow the field further and demonstrate that the virus probably reacts solely with the nerve-cell body and its processes. This is shown by the following two experiments (9, Ch. III; 12).

It is familiar to all students of neurology that interruption of a fiber

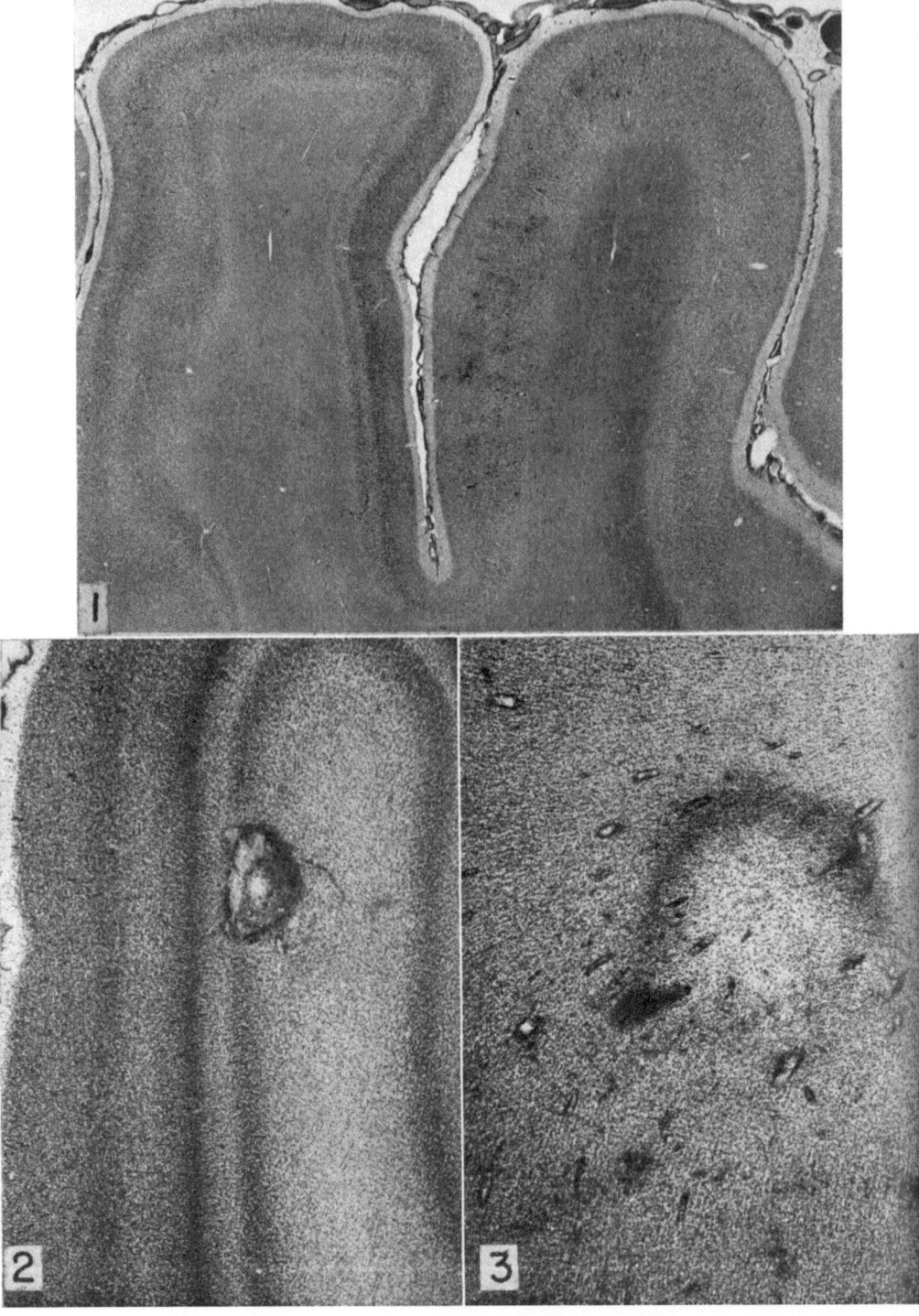

tract in the central nervous system usually leads to complete retrograde degeneration of its cells of origin. This reaction was utilized for eliminating the cells of the lateral nucleus of the thalamus by damaging their terminals in the cerebral cortex through removal of the appropriate cerebral hemisphere. Control material showed that one month after operation, there was almost complete loss of nerve cells in the lateral thalamic nucleus, with increase of glial cells in response to the regressive process. A few scattered neurons remained, but, in the main, it had been possible to obtain an area which was devoid of nerve cells but in which the supporting tissues and vascular system were not directly or seriously disturbed. Access of the virus into the prepared area was insured by direct inoculation of a potent virus suspension into it. The animals so inoculated contracted typical paralytic poliomyelitis. Lesions consisting of areas of neuronophagia, and perivascular cuffing, were seen in the normal parts of the thalamus and subthalamus, but were absent from the area which was devoid of nerve cells (Plate II, Fig. 1). It is probably significant that the only lymphocytic reaction in this area occurred directly around the inoculum, which was composed of a spinal-cord emulsion containing not only virus but the debris of cells destroyed by the virus. These findings make it reasonably clear that the characteristic cellular responses seen in poliomyelitis—namely, focal infiltrations of leucocytes and perivascular cuffs—are called into being by the reaction of the virus with neurons and with neurons only, since the reaction did not appear in areas devoid of neurons.

While there is abundant evidence to show that virus is disseminated

---

PLATE I

FIGURE 1. CASE H12. HUMAN PARALYTIC POLIOMYELITIS. LEFT CEREBRAL CORTEX, SHOWING THE CENTRAL SULCUS (CENTER)
Note lesions in precentral (motor) cortex and their absence from postcentral cortex. Gallocyanin. Magnification = × 5.

FIGURE 2. RHESUS 548. OCCIPITAL POLE (AREA 17 OF BRODMANN) WITH POTENT VIRUS-CONTAINING INOCULUM
Note the absence of response of mesodermal-glial tissues in this region of the cortex. Gallocyanin. Magnification = × 21.

FIGURE 3. RHESUS 691. MOTOR CORTEX (AREA 4)
Note the abundance of lesions, perivascular and focal, which occurs in this susceptible region of the cortex surrounding the inoculum. Gallocyanin. Magnification = × 21.

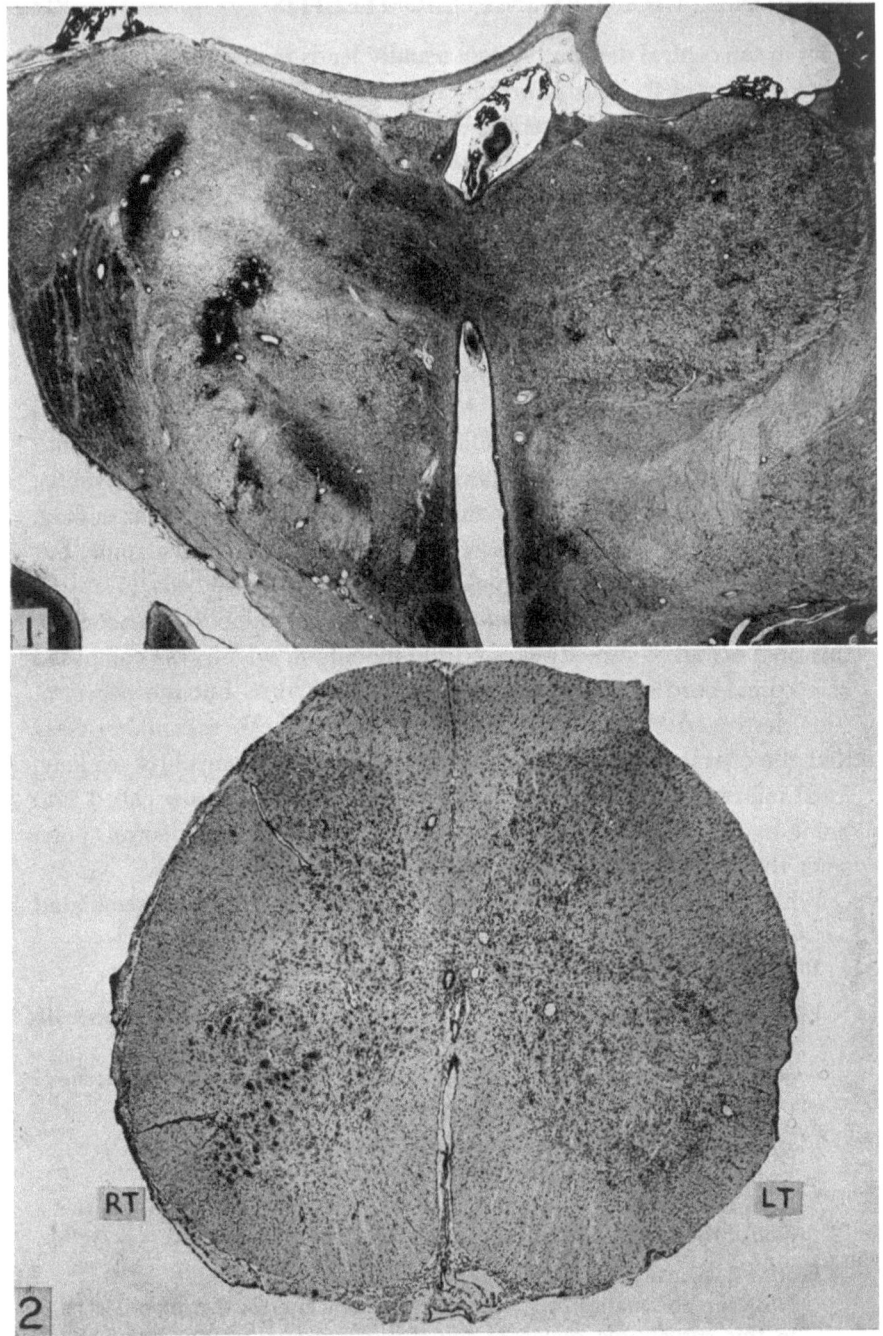

through the nervous system along nerve pathways, rather than by diffuse extension through the supporting tissues, it has been difficult to obtain definite information as to the precise nervous elements which are involved in this process. A very different approach has been employed to accumulate data on this point (9, Ch. II; 13). In this case, advantage was taken of the fact that regenerating anterior horn cells become refractory to poliomyelitis virus (9, Ch. IX; 14). Twelve to fourteen days after section of a peripheral nerve, such as the sciatic, the cells of origin of the nerve in the anterior horn of the spinal cord become resistant to destruction by poliomyelitis virus (Plate II, Fig. 2). This refractory state persists until functional recovery of the nerve has been effected, at which time the motor cells again become normally susceptible. Three repeated sections of the sciatic nerve, at intervals of roughly two weeks, raised the threshold of the refractory cells to such a level that after the freshly cut end of the sciatic nerve was dipped into virus, infection took place in only one of six animals, whereas the same procedure produced paralysis in eleven of thirteen normal animals.[2]

The interpretation of this experiment is as follows: Section of a peripheral nerve produces changes of a widely different character in the distal and proximal segments of the nerve. Whereas typical Wallerian degeneration is seen in the former, the visible changes in the

[2] According to the chi square test, $P=.01$.

PLATE II

FIGURE 1. RHESUS A50. THALAMUS STAINED WITH TOLUIDIN BLUE
Note the severe retrograde degeneration in the ventrolateral nuclear mass and pulvinar on the left, with two deeply staining inocula placed within these centers. Focal and perivascular lesions are absent in the neuron-denuded regions containing the inocula of virus, but are numerous in the undegenerated nucleus centrum medianum, substantia nigra, and field of Forel on the left, and in the ventrolateral nuclear mass on the right. Gallocyanin. Magnification $= \times 5$.

FIGURE 2. RHESUS AO. LUMBAR CORD, SHOWING SPARING OF THE ANTERIOR HORN CELLS IN THE RIGHT SCIATIC NUCLEUS
The right sciatic nerve had been sectioned twenty-five days before virus reached the lumbar cord in destructive concentrations. Note the complete destructions of cells on the left side (right in figure). Gallocyanin. Magnification $= \times 20$.

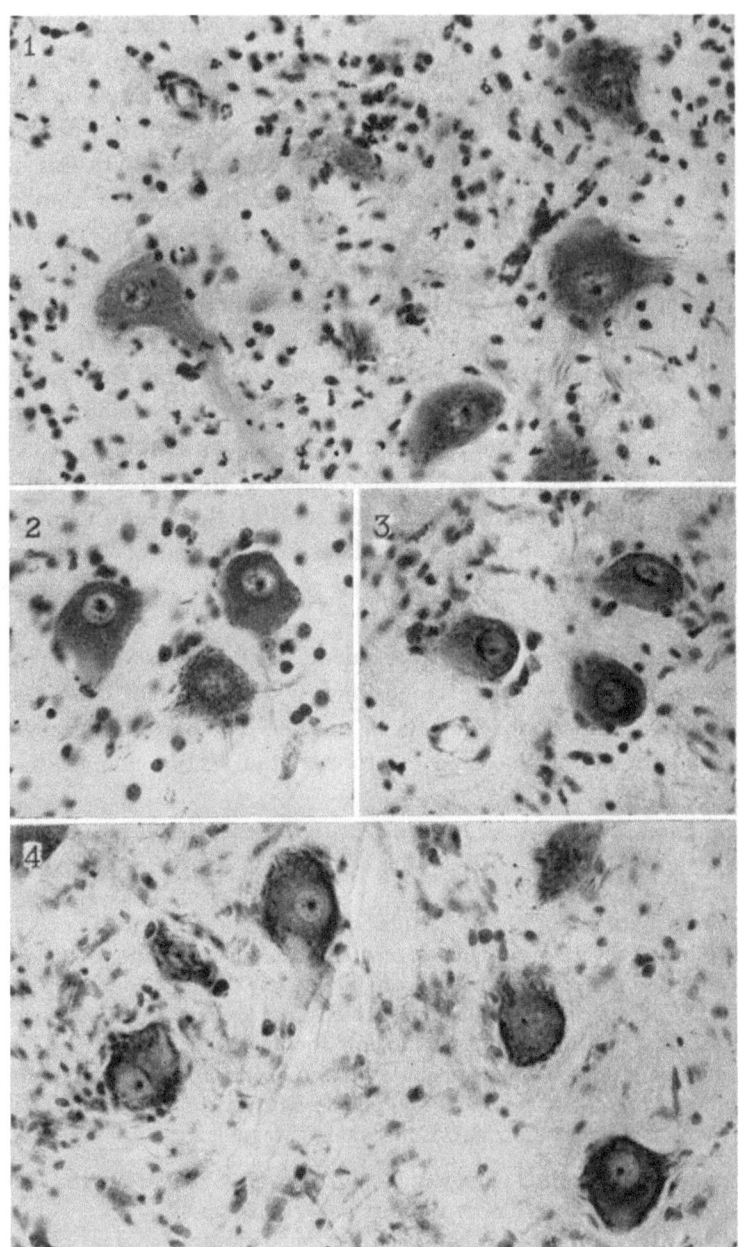

central segment are confined to the cell bodies giving rise to the axon of the nerve. These changes in the cell body associated with the development of the virus refractory state, will be described later. In this context, it is important to point out that while no changes are seen, in either the sheath or the axon of the central segment, the axons are, in fact, a part of the cytoplasm of the virus refractory cells lying within the anterior horn. Furthermore, Bodian and Flexner (15) have shown an increase in acid phosphatase activity in this segment of the nerve, as well as in the nerve-cell body. We therefore have some reason for believing that the axon may have altered properties, whereas the myelin sheath does not. The fact that direct contact between virus and axons from refractory cells fails to result in disease therefore strongly suggests that the axon, as well as the nerve-cell body, is highly selective for the virus, the former serving as a medium for its dissemination through the nervous system, and the latter as a locus at which virus titer is increased. Further corroboration of this latter conclusion is the fact that virus is much easier to demonstrate in the regions of the central nervous system containing susceptible gray matter than in peripheral nerves or in white matter.

Following the introduction of poliomyelitis virus into the brain or

PLATE III

THE PRINCIPAL MORPHOLOGICAL STAGES OF INJURED AND RECOVERING MOTONEURONS, DURING THE FIRST WEEK OF THE DISEASE
Gallocyanin. Magnification = × 250. (Reprinted by permission of the editor of the *Johns Hopkins Hospital Bulletin*.)

FIGURE 1. RHESUS B12, PREPARALYTIC PERIOD
Note the diffuse character of chromatolysis in the three motoneurons below. The one at upper right is essentially normal.

FIGURE 2. RHESUS A794, THIRD DAY AFTER ONSET OF PARALYSIS
Transitional stage, with motonuerons showing "new" granular Nissl bodies, and accumulation of Nissl substance near cell and nuclear membranes.

FIGURE 3. RHESUS B338, FIFTH DAY AFTER ONSET OF PARALYSIS
Early stage of central chromatolysis with definite membrane accumulation of Nissl substance, and pale central zone of cytoplasm.

FIGURE 4. RHESUS B935, SEVENTH DAY AFTER ONSET OF PARALYSIS
Typical central chromatolysis with "filling-in" of central cytoplasmic area by "new" Nissl bodies.

nose of a susceptible animal, the virus may be demonstrated for as long as forty-eight hours at the site of inoculation, but it then disappears (16). After a latent period of three or more days, depending upon the strain of virus used, the preparalytic period is ushered in by an elevation of temperature. Usually within one to three days neurological signs indicating central nervous system invasion appear, although paralysis does not ensue for some hours. The preparalytic period is characterized by a rapid spread of virus through the entire neuraxis. Animals sacrificed in this period, a few hours after the appearance of fever, usually show many lesions (17). Even before weakness of limbs can be detected, the virus titer in the cord has risen to a maximum, and many cells are showing histological evidence of virus invasion. The subsequent chain of events has been most clearly described in a recent paper by Bodian (18), which will form the basis of my discussion of this point.

The first visible effects of the virus upon the motoneurons is seen in the cytoplasm. It consists of beginning dissolution of the deeply basophilic Nissl bodies in the cell cytoplasm. The process, known as chromatolysis, is seen as the primary reaction of the nerve cell to various noxious stimuli, such as axon section, anoxia, toxins, and viruses. In this case it progresses to complete loss of the identity of the Nissl bodies, leaving the cytoplasm pale and diffusely blue when stained with the thiazin dyes. (Plate III, Figs. 1, 2). In the preparalytic period the majority of the cells show this diffuse chromatolysis in varying degree, although many have pycnotic nuclei and a few are frankly necrotic. Nuclear eccentricity is reatively uncommon. It may be safely concluded, at this stage of the disease, that all the changes observed are degenerative. Mild chromatolysis may be present before perivascular cuffing or cellular infiltration is apparent. In severe paralytic infections, the majority of the cells show marked diffuse chromatolysis, frank vacuolization, or neuronophagia. In cases with mild paralysis most of the cells are diffusely chromatolytic. It is important to emphasize that in examining the cord segments supplying fifty-four extremities in acute cases, Bodian found none in which more than 31 percent of the expected number of cells appeared normal. This indicates, in the monkey at least, that virus is widely disseminated, even in mild cases, and that motoneurons continue to function, even when they show definite evidence of virus invasion.

On the second and third days of paralysis there appear for the first time nerve cells apparently showing re-formation of Nissl bodies. The earliest stages show an accumulation of basophilic material, sometimes around the nucleus (Plate III, Fig. 3) but usually at the periphery of the cell (Plate III, Fig. 4). This latter cell type, showing chromatolysis only in its center, is present in large numbers by the fourth to the sixth day, at which time neuronophagia is no longer apparent and paralysis not progressive (Plate IV). By the ninth day, the cells either are normal in appearance or are showing only central chromatolysis. It is not uncommon to find normal-looking cells with acidophilic intranuclear inclusions, suggesting previous invasion with almost complete recovery.

Axon degeneration is not seen until at least two and one-half days after the onset of paralysis. It is of further interest that in spinal-cord segments which show severe chromatolysis but little frank necrosis of neurons, the axons retain their normal appearance.

By the third week less than 10 percent of the surviving neurons are abnormal in appearance. While there are a few bizarre forms, the majority of these abnormal cells show central chromatolysis. Bodian has quantitated this entire cycle by counts of the numbers of the motor cells in the anterior horns of the limb regions, both in normal monkeys and in those exhibiting all stages of paralysis and recovery. It is evident from his data that all the destruction of cells takes place during the first three days of paralysis. From this point the numbers of normal and abnormal cells vary in inverse ratio, thus forcing the conclusion that "the increase in normal cells after the 2nd to 5th days, must occur by the recovery of abnormal cells."

The facts so far presented, indicate the high selectivity of poliomyelitis virus for certain neurons in the central nervous system. It is also evident that the visible degenerative and regenerative changes in the neurons correspond very closely in time with the easily observed cycle of paralysis and recovery in the experimental animal, thus rendering it unnecessary to postulate an important role for inflammation or edema in the etiology of paralysis.

The observation that motoneurons become refractory to virus during axonal regeneration (9, Ch. IX; 14) has offered the very intriguing opportunity of investigating the metabolic changes which underlie this altered physiological state (Plate V). The conditions appear to be

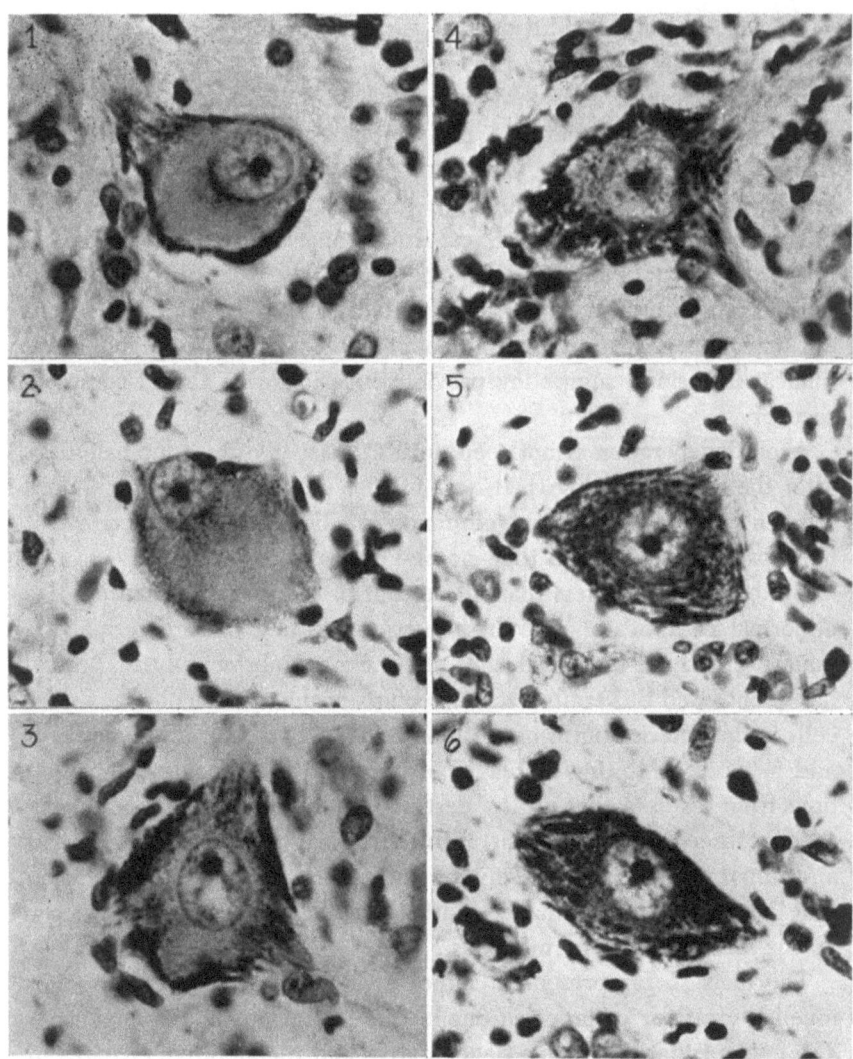

very favorable for such a study because one is dealing with a group of cells which do not divide and which may be influenced by events (namely, axon section) in the periphery which do not disturb the spinal cord. A further advantage is found in the fact that only the neurons participate in the experimental procedure and that one anterior horn of the same animal can be used as a control.

In the beginning an effort was made to relate the development of the virus refractory state to the well-known histological phenomenon of chromatolysis. On this latter subject there exists an enormous literature, which need not be summarized here. Suffice it to say that axon section induces a "lysis" of the chromophilic material (Nissl bodies) in the cytoplasm of the nerve cell (19). Within seven to ten days, depending upon the proximity of the section to the nerve-cell body, there is dissolution of the Nissl bodies in the cytoplasm of the nerve cell, which becomes pale and homogeneous when stained with basic dyes. The nucleus becomes markedly eccentric. Regrowth of the axon is accompanied by a reversal of these changes. Nissl bodies contain protein and ribose nucleic acid (20), and at first, since the virus, by analogy with others (21), is thought also to contain nucleic acid of some kind, it was very tempting to consider the Nissl bodies as an immediate substrate for virus growth. It turned out, however, that the period of maximal resistance to virus came some days later than that of maximal Nissl body reduction, and persisted into a period when protein synthesis, as judged by reformation of Nissl bodies, was well advanced. It therefore appeared that the virus refractory state depended upon events more complexly determined even than the histologically visible changes in the nerve-cell body. What initial hypotheses could one entertain? Did the virus fail to enter the cell because of membrane changes? This hypothesis may be discarded because it was found that cells rendered chromatolytic by axon section became more

---

PLATE IV

CHIMPANZEE A434, SEVENTH DAY AFTER ONSET OF PARALYSIS
Gallocyanin. Magnification = × 480. (Reprinted by permission of the editors of the *Journal of Experimental Medicine*.)

FIGURES 1 to 6 show a group of cells arranged in the sequence of increasing recovery from the chromatolysis of the acute stage.

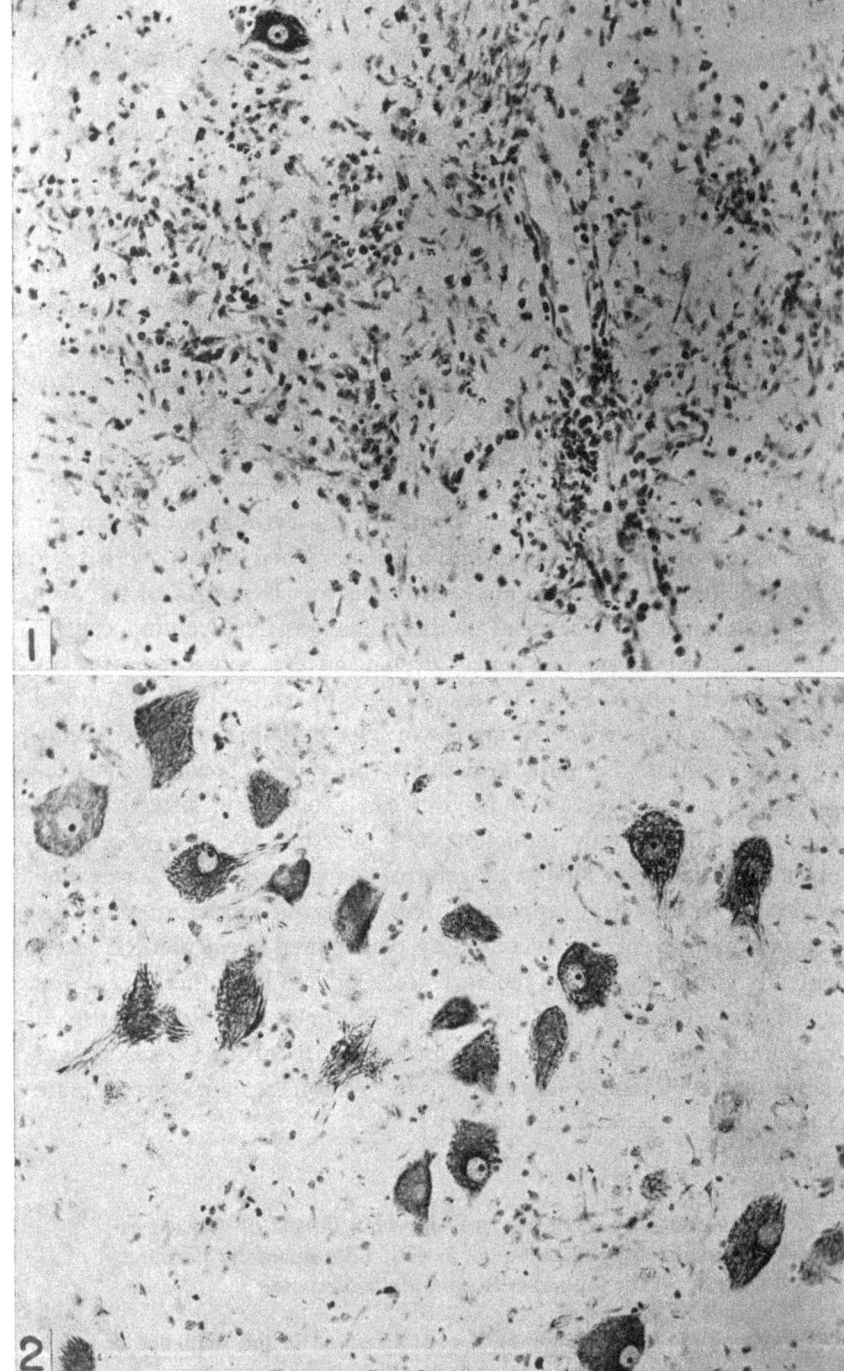

so after exposure to virus, and also contained acidophilic intranuclear inclusions. Was it possible that the virus failed to propagate because of unfavorable energy relations within the cell? A valuable pilot experiment bearing upon the latter would have been a study of aerobic and anaerobic glycolysis to determine any over-all alteration in cell metabolism. This turned out to be impossible with the techniques then at our disposal, because of the peculiar anatomical constitution of the central nervous system. It must be recalled that the cells of the anterior horn represent a small fraction of the tissue constituting the spinal cord, and that changes in these small elements must be measured in the presence of a relatively large amounts of tissue which does not participate in the reaction to peripheral nerve section. For example, after section of all the lumbosacral or cervical nerve roots at the plexus levels, consistent differences in aerobic glycolysis between the normal and operated sides could not be detected in tissue slices. Attempts to isolate the anterior horns by dissection were scarcely more successful, since it was found that after manipulation, the O_2 consumption of the two anterior horns of a normal cord varied as widely as that observed in experimental material.

In the end we were forced to use a method which could eliminate all tissue except the gray matter of the anterior horn and which at the same time gave consistent results in the controls. This involved exposure of the cord in the living, anesthetized animal, its rapid removal with freezing on dry ice, triming away of all extraneous white matter, and final emulsification of the isolated anterior horn. Since we were not able to detect any glycolytic activity with our methods, it was

---

PLATE V

FIGURE 1. RHESUS A28. LEFT ANTERIOR HORN OF THE LUMBAR CORD (CONTROL SIDE), SHOWING COMPLETE DESTRUCTION OF THE MOTOR CELLS
Gallocyanin. Magnification = × 175.

FIGURE 2. RHESUS A28. RIGHT ANTERIOR HORN OF THE LUMBAR CORD, SHOWING SPARING OF MOTOR CELLS IN THE RIGHT SCIATIC NUCLEUS
The right sciatic nerve had been sectioned ninety-one days previous to paralysis. Note that the Nissl bodies have nearly recovered their normal size (compare with the single normal cell in Fig. 1) but that the nuclei are still eccentric.

necessary to turn to some enzyme system which was relatively resistant to freezing and homogenation, even although it represented only a part of the total oxidative mechanism of the cell. The first studies were therefore begun on the succinoxidase system and have been carried out in collaboration with Dr. Robert Mellors (22) and Dr. Josefa Flexner (23). Since these have already been published and the techniques described in full, I shall merely mention the findings here. Suffice it to say that we used the manometric methods of Stotz (24) for cytochrome oxidase, and those of Schneider and Potter (25) and Quastel and Wheatley (26) for succinic dehydrogenase. The experimental findings were rigidly controlled by calculation of the sampling variation encountered in the corresponding sides of the central nervous system of normal animals.

Before beginning the study of regenerating motoneurons it was imperative also to get some idea of the sensitivity of the method. For this purpose, we utilized the deneuronated thalamus preparation already described, studying cytochrome oxidase in the normal thalamus of the cat, and in that from which the neurons had been brought to degeneration by decortication a month previously. Virtually complete subtraction of the thalamic neurons resulted in a 35 percent reduction of cytochrome oxidase activity (Table 1). Similarly, studies of succinic

TABLE 1[a]

CYTOCHROME OXIDASE UNITS IN THALAMUS (CAT)

	CONTROL SERIES				EXPERIMENTAL SERIES				
Experiment	Right	Left	Difference	Percent Difference	Experiment	Normal	Deneuronated	Difference[b]	Percent Difference
68	4.44	4.97	+0.53	+11	54	5.24	4.05	−1.19	−23
69, 70	5.03	6.38	+1.35	+21	64	6.15	5.15	−1.00	−16
71, 72	6.78	6.80	+0.02	+3	65	7.38	4.31	−3.07	−42
73	6.75	6.43	−0.32	−5	81	5.10	2.70	−2.40	−47
89	4.88	5.04	+0.16	+3	82	5.45	2.93	−2.52	−46
90	4.60	4.52	−0.08	−2					
92	4.11	5.03	+0.92	+18					
Mean	5.22	5.59	+0.37	+7	Mean	5.86	3.84	−2.04	−35
Sigma mean difference			0.21		Sigma mean difference			0.45	

[a] Reprinted by permission of the editors of the *Journal of Experimental Medicine*.
[b] This column represents the cytochrome oxidase activity of the thalamic neurones.

dehydrogenase activity, by the method of Schneider and Potter, showed an average reduction of 41 percent in the anterior horns of monkeys in which virtually all of the motoneurons had been destroyed

TABLE 2[a]

SUCCINIC DEHYDROGENASE IN MONKEY ANTERIOR HORN; COMPARISON OF POLIOMYELITIC AND NORMAL CORDS

	METHOD OF SCHNEIDER AND POTTER QO_2 (SUCCINATE)[b]				METHOD OF QUASTEL AND WHEATLEY $\Delta Q \; {}^{N_2}_{CO_2}$ (SUCCINATE)[c]	
No Muscle Function	5–50 Percent Muscle Function	70–80 Percent Muscle Function	Normal		0–40 Percent Muscle Function	Normal
2.20	2.16	2.92	Average		3.41	Average
2.23	2.35	3.05	of 41		4.41	of 17
2.31	2.59	3.20	anterior		4.77	anterior
2.33	2.70	3.33	horns		5.05	horns
2.35	2.71	3.56			5.24	
2.37	2.80	3.71			5.29	
2.94	2.94	3.74			5.66	
	2.94				6.12	
	3.48					
Mean 2.39	2.74	3.36	4.07		4.87	8.42
% below normal 41	33	17	0		40	0
Difference between groups σ	2.4	3.7	5.6		3	

[a] Reprinted by permission of the editors of the *Journal of Biological Chemistry*.
[b] C.mm. of O_2 per hour per mg. (wet weight) of tissue.
[c] C.mm. of CO_2 per hour per mg. (wet weight) of tissue.

by poliomyelitis (Table 2). It was therefore probable that at least large changes in the activity of these enzymes within the neurons could be measured in the presence of activity in the supporting tissues and blood vessels. At the same time it was indicated that, since the nerve cells represent a small part of the total volume of the thalamus or anterior horn (possibly 1/50 in the latter case), but contribute 35 to 40 percent of its activity, the enzyme activity of nerve tissue must be considerably higher than that of supporting tissues.

When the succinoxidase system was investigated in the anterior

TABLE 3[a]

CYTOCHROME OXIDASE UNITS IN ANTERIOR HORN OF MONKEY SPINAL CORD

CONTROL SERIES					EXPERIMENTAL SERIES 7–9 days				
Experiment	Right	Left	Difference	Percent Difference	Experiment	Right	Left	Difference	Percent Difference
509	0.88	0.92	+0.04	+4	722	0.77	0.77	0	0
575	0.50	0.64	+0.14	+21	800	1.03	1.03	−0.09	−8
588–9	0.58	0.72	+0.14	+19	810	0.91	0.89	−0.02	−2
718	0.41	0.37	−0.04	−9	811	0.62	0.64	+0.02	+3
720	0.64	0.67	+0.03	+5	828	0.88	0.77	−0.10	−11
723	1.01	1.01	0	0	833	0.52	0.56	+0.04	+7
740	0.40	0.44	+0.04	+9					
748	0.52	0.51	−0.01	−2	Mean	0.80	0.77	−0.03	−3.75
754	0.55	0.59	+0.04	−7	Sigma mean difference			0.02	
767	0.81	0.73	−0.08	−10					
Mean	0.63	0.66	+0.03	+4.5	10–20 days				
Sigma mean difference			0.02		383	0.69	0.35	−0.34	−49
					499	0.97	0.66	−0.31	−32
					500	0.65	0.64	−0.01	−2
					562	0.64	0.67	+0.03	+5
					541[b]	1.52	0.60	−0.92	−61
					813	0.74	0.73	−0.01	−1
					Mean	0.74	0.61	−0.13	−17.5
					Sigma mean difference			0.14	
					21 days and over[c]				
					504	0.66	0.42	−0.24	−36
					645	0.47	0.48	+0.01	+2
					646	0.75	0.62	−0.13	−17
					682	0.53	0.45	−0.08	−15
					683	1.00	0.74	−0.26	−26
					687	0.36	0.24	−0.12	−33
					Mean	0.63	0.49	−0.14	−22
					Sigma mean difference			0.04	

[a] Reprinted by permission of the editors of the *Journal of Experimental Medicine*.

[b] This reading, which is obviously out of line, was omitted in calculating the mean, but was included in the calculation of sigma.

[c] The probability that by chance alone in 5 of 6 tests, the figure for the left side would be lower than that for the right by 15 per cent or more is one in a hundred.

horns, following section of the limb plexuses or spinal roots on one side, it was found that for the first week after nerve section, there was little change from the normal values (Tables 3, 4). Similarly, at this

TABLE 4[a]

QO_2 (SUCCINATE)[b] OF ANTERIOR HORN OF MONKEY SPINAL CORD FOLLOWING NERVE SECTION

7 DAYS				10–12 DAYS				32–54 DAYS			
Experiment	Normal	Operated	Percent Difference	Experiment	Normal	Operated	Percent Difference	Experiment	Normal	Operated	Percent Difference
B681	4.59	4.20	−8.5	B270	4.09	3.58	−12.5	B169	3.69	3.41	−7.6
B682	5.14	5.28	+2.7	B271	3.89	3.74	−3.9	A999	3.71	3.31	−10.8
B708	4.57	4.47	−2.3	B272	4.12	3.82	−7.9	B53	4.33	4.14	−4.4
B709	3.92	3.88	−1.0	B296	4.63	4.20	−9.3	B192	3.87	3.20	17.3
B744	4.52	4.35	−3.8	B722	4.14	3.79	−8.6	B193	4.02	3.37	−15.4
B745	4.50	4.27	−5.1	B723	4.48	4.15	−7.4	B194	4.51	4.01	−11.1
				B747	4.37	4.13	−5.5	B195	4.11	3.61	−12.2
								B219	3.98	3.35	−15.8
								B220	3.83	3.42	−10.8
								B221	4.29	3.70	−13.8
Mean	4.54	4.41	−2.9		4.25	3.91	−7.8		4.03	3.55	−11.9
σ of mean			1.44				0.97				1.25
				$\dfrac{x}{\sigma} = 7.2$				$\dfrac{x}{\sigma} = 8.4$			

[a] Reprinted by permission of the editors of the *Journal of Biological Chemistry*.
[b] C.mm. of O_2 per hour per mg. (wet weight) of tissue.

period there was no evidence that the cells had become virus-refractory. At ten to twenty-one days, when the virus-refractory state is first established, succinoxidase levels were significantly depressed, while at twenty-one to fifty days, when the virus-refractory state is maximal, a depression of 22 percent of cytochrome oxidase activity and 12 percent of succinic dehydrogenase, was observed. Since the activity of the anterior horn was known, both with and without motoneurons, data were at hand to calculate that an over-all reduction of 12 percent in the anterior horn represented a reduction of approximately 30 percent in the individual neurons.

Bodian and Mellors (27) were able to show that nerve-root section induced an average decrease of 43 percent in the phosphocreatine of the anterior horn on the operated side (Table 5). Although their work

TABLE 5[a]

PHOSPHOCREATINE IN ANTERIOR HORN OF MONKEY SPINAL CORD
The values are expressed in mg. of P per 100 gm. of tissue

CONTROL SERIES					EXPERIMENTAL SERIES				
Experiment No.	Normal Left	Normal Right	Difference	Percent Difference	Experiment No.	Regenerating Left	Normal Right	Difference	Percent Difference
Cervical cord									
A717	18.2	16.8	+1.4	+7.7	A738	5.6	7.4	−1.8	−24.3
A719	9.7	10.2	−0.5	−4.9	A739	4.3	8.0	−3.7	−46.4
A754	5.8	6.2	−0.4	−6.5	A797	12.5	10.9	+1.6	+14.5
A730	16.6	15.2	+1.4	+8.4	A778	8.9	20.6	−11.7	−56.7
A667	12.8	10.6	+2.2	+17.2	A779	4.6	16.8	−12.2	−72.0
A777	13.7	14.4	−0.7	−4.9	A780	6.1	31.8	−25.7	−81.0
A806	14.3	14.0	+0.3	+2.1	A677	5.0	15.9	−10.9	−68.6
A774	22.9	14.2	+8.7	+38.0	A684	18.0	22.6	−4.6	−20.4
A773	7.9	10.1	−2.2	−21.8	A559	9.8	17.6	−7.8	−44.3
					A688	10.6	15.2	−4.6	−30.2
Lumbar cord									
A717	23.2	19.0	+4.2	+18.2	A738	11.5	16.3	−4.8	−29.4
A754	7.1	5.9	+1.2	+16.9	A739	3.6	4.8	−1.2	−25.0
A730	29.5	26.4	+3.1	+10.5	A797	15.2	16.3	−1.1	−6.8
A667	21.7	20.7	+1.0	+4.6	A778	8.1	9.9	−1.8	−18.2
A777	12.7	12.5	+0.2	+1.6	A779	6.3	14.2	−7.9	−55.5
A806	8.4	7.8	+0.6	+7.2	A780	16.6	29.2	−12.6	−43.1
					A802	13.1	22.4	−9.3	−41.4
Mean	15.0	13.6	+1.37	+9.1		9.4	16.5	−7.1	−43.0
σ mean difference			0.64					1.53	

[a] Reprinted by permission of the editors of the *Journal of Biological Chemistry*.

was interrupted by the war, they at least obtained this one suggestion that this energy-rich phosphorus compound might be deficient under the conditions of the experiment.

I shall now attempt a synthesis of these quite meager facts—perhaps even a projection into speculation. We are now fairly sure that in the central nervous system, the virus multiplies only in the nerve cell and its processes. The amazing specificity of the virus, not only for certain animal species but also for particular types of nerve cells in a particular host, suggests that some characteristic protein is important in the synthesis of virus. Yet, anterior horn cells are still susceptible to virus at a time when the protein and pentose nucleic acid of the Nissl bodies has been strikingly reduced by root section. It is during the period of re-formation of Nissl bodies that motoneurons become refractory to virus. This argues, then, that the protein of the Nissl bodies is not incorporated directly into virus protein or that it may lack some essential constituent for many weeks.

The succinoxidase and phosphocreatine studies indicate altered cell metabolism in the direction of reduction. We do not at the moment have the data to know whether this is part of an over-all reduction, or one involving only certain systems. The observed changes are the concomitant of an apparent adjustment of the cell to a smaller volume but a presumably increased growth demand. This suggests a return of the nerve cell to a quasi-embryonic state, and it may not be irrelevant that both regenerating nerve cells, as well as regenerating liver cells (28), when compared with normal cells from the same animal, appear to show certain features in common. While liver cells undergo mitosis and nerve cells do not, there is, nevertheless, a growth phase which may be comparable in the two. At any rate, both show an increase in pentose nucleic acid which is doubtless of cytoplasmic origin. There is a concomitant low level of succinoxidase activity in both cell types, with the additional finding of reduced activity for malic dehydrogenase, cytochrome reductase, and oxalacetic oxidase in the regenerating liver. These findings suggest a diversion of cellular metabolism to other and possibly less efficient pathways. Certainly it would be going far beyond the available data to more than hazard that the available cellular energy may not be sufficient for the synthesis of both Nissl-body nucleoprotein and virus protein. Under these conditions the virus may be ineffectual in the competition for substrate, and unable to establish the diversion of protein synthesis which would favor virus production and at the same time lead to the death of the cell.

SUMMARY

This review is an attempt to collect various lines of evidence for the strictly neuronotropic character of poliomyelitis virus and to point out some of the problems connected with the study of the ways in which the virus and the susceptible nerve cell interact with one another. It represents largely the work of one group which has extended over a period of more than ten years and which has not been collected in precisely this manner before. As the paper itself is almost a telegraphic summary, it seems valueless to make a further condensation of it.

REFERENCES

1. Di Vesta, A., and G. Zagari, La transmission de la rage par voie nerveuse, *Ann. de L'Inst. Pasteur*, 1889, 3:237.
2. Schweinburg, F., and F. Windholz, Über den Ausbreitungsweg des Wuterregers von der Eintrittspforte aus, *Virchows Arch. f. Path. Anat.*, 1930, 278:23.
3. Hurst, E. W., Infection of the rhesus monkey (Macaca mulatta) and the guinea-pig with the virus of equine encephalomyelitis, *J. Path. & Bact.*, 1936, 42:271.
4. Haymaker, Webb, A. B. Sabin, Topographic distribution of lesions in the central nervous system in Japanese B encephalitis, *Arch. Neurol. & Psychiat.*, 1947, 57:673.
5. Thomas, L., and J. L. Peck, Results of inoculating Okinawan horses with the virus of Japanese B encephalitis, *Proc. Soc. Exp. Biol. & Med.*, 1946, 61:5.
6. Smithburn, K. C., T. P. Hughes, A. W. Burke, and J. H. Paul, A neurotropic virus isolated from the blood of a native of Uganda, *Am. J. Trop. Med.*, 1940, 20:471.
7. Kling, C., W. Wernstedt, and A. Petterson, Recherches sur le mode de propogation de la paralysis infantile épidémique (maladie de Heine-Medin), *Ztschr. f. Immunitätsforschung*, 1912, 12:316.
8. Howe, H. A., and D. Bodian, Poliomyelitis in the chimpanzee: a clinical pathological study, *Bull. Johns Hopkins Hosp.*, 1941, 69:149.
9. Howe, H. A., and D. Bodian, Neural Mechanisms in Poliomyelitis (New York, 1942).
10. Howe, H. A., and D. Bodian, Neuropathological evidence on the portal of entry problem in human poliomyelitis, *Bull. Johns Hopkins Hosp.*, 1941, 69:183.
11. Bodian, D., and H. A. Howe, An experimental study of the role of neurones in the dissemination of poliomyelitis virus in the nervous system, *Brain*, 1940, 63:135.
12. Bodian, D., and H. A. Howe, Neurotropism and the genesis of cerebral lesions in poliomyelitis, an experimental study, *Bull. Johns Hopkins Hosp.*, 1941, 68:58.
13. Bodian, D., and H. A. Howe, Experimental studies on intraneural spread of poliomyelitis virus, *Bull. Johns Hopkins Hosp.*, 1941, 68:248.
14. Howe, H. A., and D. Bodian, Refractoriness of nerve cells to poliomyelitis virus after interruption of their axones, *Bull. Johns Hopkins Hosp.*, 1941, 69:92.
15. Bodian, D., Nucleic acid in nerve cell regeneration. Symposia of Soc. Exp. Biol., No. 1, *Nucleic Acid*, pp. 163–178 (Cambridge, 1947).

16. Sabin, A. B., and P. K. Olitsky, Fate of nasally instilled poliomyelitis virus in normal and convalescent monkeys with special reference to the problem of host to host transmission, *J. Exp. Med.*, 1938, 68:39.
17. Bodian, D., and M. C. Cumberland, The rise and decline of poliomyelitis virus levels in infected nervous tissue, *Am. J. Hyg.*, 1947, 45:226.
18. Bodian, D., The virus, the nerve cell, and paralysis: A study of experimental poliomyelitis in the spinal cord, *Bull. Johns Hopkins Hosp.*, 1948, 83:1.
19. Nissl, F., Die Beziehungen der Nervenzellensubstanzer zu den thätigen, ruhenden, und ermüdeten Zellzuständen, *Allg. Ztschr. f. Psychiat.*, 1896, 52:1147.
20. Gersch, I., and D. Bodian, Some chemical mechanisms in chromatolysis, *J. Cell. & Comp. Physiol.*, 1943, 21:253.
21. Beard, J. W., Review: Purified Animal Viruses, *J. Immunol.*, 1948, 58:49.
22. Howe, H. A., and R. C. Mellors, Cytochrome oxidase in normal and regenerating neurons, *J. Exp. Med.*, 1945, 81:489.
23. Howe, H. A., and J. B. Flexner, Succinic dehydrogenase in regenerating neurons, *J. Biol. Chem.*, 1947, 167:663.
24. Stotz, E., The estimation and distribution of cytochrome oxidase and cytochrome C in rat tissues, *J. Biol. Chem.*, 1939, 131:555.
25. Schneider, W. C., and V. R. Potter, The assay of animal tissues for respiratory enzymes, II: Succinic dehydrogenase and cytochrome oxidase, *J. Biol. Chem.*, 1943, 149:217.
26. Quastel, J. H., and A. H. M. Wheatley, Anaerobic oxidations. On ferricyanide as a reagent for the manometric investigation of dehydrogenase systems, *Biochem. J.*, 1938, 32:936.
27. Bodian, D., and R. C. Mellors, Decrease of phosphocreatine in regenerating neurons, *J. Biol. Chem.*, 1947, 167:655.
28. Novikoff, A. B., and Van R. Potter, Biochemical studies on regenerating liver, *J. Biol. Chem.*, 1947, 173:223.

SYMPOSIA OF
THE SECTION ON MICROBIOLOGY
THE NEW YORK ACADEMY OF MEDICINE

1. Diagnosis of Viral and Rickettsial Infections
   Edited by Frank L. Horsfall, Jr.

2. Evaluation of Chemotherapeutic Agents
   Edited by Colin M. MacLeod

3. The Pathogenesis and Pathology of Viral Diseases
   Edited by John G. Kidd

Bei Fragen zur Produktsicherheit wenden Sie sich bitte an:
If you have any questions regarding product safety,
please contact:

Walter de Gruyter GmbH
Genthiner Straße 13
10785 Berlin
productsafety@degruyterbrill.com